The Coconut Plant: Pathways to Health and Wellness

HERBAL HEALTH, Volume 3

Mogana S. Flomo, Jr.

Published by CEPRES International University, 2025.

THE COCONUT PLANT: PATHWAYS TO HEALTH AND WELLNESS

First edition. October 28, 2025.

ISBN: 979-8232558802

Written by Mogana S. Flomo, Jr..

Also by Mogana S. Flomo, Jr.

First Edition

Introduction to University Studies

Rethinking PhD Training: A 21st Century Approach

HERBAL HEALTH

The Miracle of Bryophyllum pinnatum

The Coconut Plant: Pathways to Health and Wellness

Standalone

Food and Drug Interactions: A Guide for the Health worker and Patient

A Comprehensive Guide to Food Supplements

Collaboration and Knowledge Sharing in Armyworm Management

The Impact of Malaria on the Social-Economic Development of West Africa

Transforming Healthcare: Understanding Mobile Health Services in Underdeveloped Nations

Sustainable Approaches for Bird Conservation in Rice Farming: A Comprehensive Guide

Over-the-Counter (OTC) Medications: Your Comprehensive Guide to Safe and Effective Self-Care

Rejection: Embracing It and Using It

Understanding Environmental and Public Health Laws in Liberia

Understanding the National Commission on Higher Education in Liberia

School Human Resource Management

Gateways to Tomorrow: The Ultimate Admissions Guide

Integrated Disease Surveillance and Response (IDSR) in Africa

A Democratic Government: Understanding the System and Its Interconnected Parts

Short Notes On Water And Sanitation Management

Blacology

Table of Contents

"From root to crown, the coconut stands as nature's complete design—a single tree nourishing body, mind, and earth alike."

— Prof. Mogana S. Flomo, Jr.

Description

The Coconut Plant: Pathways to Health and Wellness provides an in-depth scientific and practical analysis of the coconut (*Cocos nucifera L.*) as a cornerstone of tropical nutrition and natural health. It explores the biochemical composition, nutrient density, and therapeutic potential of each component of the plant—roots, leaves, bark, flowers, and fruit—linking traditional uses with contemporary evidence from nutrition and health sciences.

Written by Prof. Mogana S. Flomo, Jr., the book emphasizes the coconut's role in promoting metabolic balance, immune resilience, cardiovascular health, and skin vitality. Drawing on ethnobotanical data and current research, it integrates holistic nutrition principles with modern dietary science to demonstrate how coconut-derived foods, oils, and beverages support optimal health.

Beyond nutritional analysis, the text presents recipes, practical applications, and wellness models that illustrate how coconut products can be incorporated into balanced diets and preventive health strategies. Intended for nutritionists, public health professionals, students, and wellness practitioners, this book bridges the gap between traditional food systems and evidence-based nutrition, positioning the coconut plant as a functional and sustainable resource for global health advancement.

Preface

For centuries, the coconut tree has stood tall and unyielding across tropical coastlines — a symbol of nourishment, resilience, and renewal. To many, it is more than a plant; it is life itself. Every part of this extraordinary tree, from its deep roots that drink from the earth to its crown of green leaves swaying against the sky, provides sustenance, healing, and protection. It is for this reason that the coconut has long been honored as "The Tree of Life."

My journey with the coconut began not as a researcher, but as an observer of how deeply it is woven into the rhythm of daily living — in food, health, tradition, and livelihood. In many communities across Africa, Asia, and the Pacific, the coconut is part of family remedies, sacred rituals, and household recipes. The wisdom surrounding this tree has been passed from generation to generation, yet much of it remains undocumented, undervalued, or forgotten in the rush of modernization.

This book was written to bring that wisdom to light — to combine tradition with science, culture with practice, and health with sustainability. It is my hope that readers will not only appreciate the coconut's many benefits but will also rediscover the connection between nature and well-being.

From its roots that heal to its fruit that nourishes, from its leaves that protect to its oil that restores — the coconut teaches us that nature provides everything we need when we learn to look closely and use it wisely.

May this work inspire a deeper respect for the natural world, and may every reader find in these pages a renewed appreciation for the divine design embedded in the Tree of Life.

— Dr. Mogana S. Flomo, Jr.

Gbarnga, Liberia

Introduction

Few plants in the natural world match the versatility of the coconut tree (Cocos nucifera). It is a single organism with a thousand uses — a source of food, water, shelter, medicine, beauty, and industry. Across continents and cultures, from the coastal villages of Liberia to the tropical islands of the Pacific, the coconut has sustained human life for centuries.

In many languages, its name translates to "giver of all that is needed." The coconut's symbolism extends beyond physical nourishment; it represents wholeness, resilience, and abundance. In traditional societies, the coconut is used in birth rituals, weddings, and religious ceremonies, signifying purity and prosperity. Its round, layered fruit has often been seen as a metaphor for life itself — hard to crack, yet filled with sweetness and strength within.

A Plant of Science and Spirit

MODERN SCIENCE CONTINUES to uncover what ancient healers already knew: that every part of the coconut holds immense health value. Its roots, bark, leaves, flowers, and fruit each contain bioactive compounds that promote healing, boost immunity, and sustain energy. Coconut oil, once dismissed as an ordinary fat, is now celebrated for its antiviral, antibacterial, and metabolic benefits. Coconut water, long treasured as a natural rehydration drink, has even been used in medical emergencies as a substitute for intravenous fluids.

Yet beyond its chemistry lies its spirit — a reminder of nature's design for harmony and interdependence. The coconut tree thrives on coastlines, bending with the wind, drinking from saltwater, and yet producing the sweetest water known to humankind. It endures where others perish, teaching lessons in resilience and adaptation.

Purpose of This Book

THIS BOOK EXPLORES the coconut in its fullness — not merely as a fruit but as a living pharmacy, a kitchen companion, and a guide to sustainable wellness. Through research, recipes, and do-it-yourself (DIY) projects, you will learn how to use every part of the coconut for health, beauty, and home living.

Each chapter blends traditional wisdom, scientific validation, and practical application — offering herbal remedies, nutritional recipes, beauty care formulas, and eco-friendly home uses. You will also encounter inspiring stories and cultural insights that reveal how deeply the coconut is embedded in human civilization.

Whether you are a health enthusiast, a herbalist, a homemaker, or simply someone seeking to reconnect with nature, this book will show you how the coconut can become a daily partner in wellness and creativity.

A Journey Through Nature's Pharmacy

AS YOU MOVE FROM CHAPTER to chapter — from the roots to the fruit, from the oil to the milk — you will discover that nothing in the coconut tree is wasted. Like life itself, it reminds us that every part has purpose, and every season brings renewal.

Welcome to the journey. Welcome to The Tree of Life.

1: The Miracle of Cocos nucifera

1.1 Origins and Identity of the Coconut Tree

Standing tall along tropical shorelines, with its slender trunk and feathery crown, the coconut tree (Cocos nucifera) has long fascinated both scientists and ordinary people. To many cultures, it is not just a tree—it is a way of life, a source of survival, and a symbol of divine providence. Its name itself tells a story: Cocos is derived from the old Portuguese and Spanish word for "monkey face," referring to the three "eyes" or depressions on the coconut shell, while nucifera means "nut-bearing." Together, Cocos nucifera means "nut-bearing coconut."

The coconut belongs to the palm family (Arecaceae), one of the oldest plant families on Earth. Fossil evidence suggests that palms have existed for more than 80 million years, and the coconut itself is thought to have originated around the Indo-Pacific region, spreading naturally across tropical coastlines by ocean currents. The fruit's remarkable ability to float and remain viable for months allowed it to travel vast distances, taking root wherever the conditions were favorable.

Today, the coconut thrives in over 90 tropical countries, from the Pacific Islands and Southeast Asia to Africa, the Caribbean, and Latin America. In Liberia and across West Africa, the coconut's presence along coastal belts tells a story of trade, migration, and adaptation — a story interwoven with human civilization itself.

1.2 The Botanical Marvel

THE COCONUT TREE IS truly a masterpiece of design. It grows up to 30 meters (about 100 feet) tall and can live for more than 60 years under favorable conditions. Its root system is fibrous, spreading widely and deeply to stabilize the tree against strong winds and coastal erosion — a natural engineering marvel. Unlike many other trees, the coconut has no taproot; instead, it develops a dense network of thousands of small roots, each absorbing water and nutrients efficiently.

The trunk, or stem, is strong yet flexible, enabling it to bend gracefully in stormy weather. This flexibility symbolizes resilience — a theme that reappears throughout this book. The leaves, known as fronds, can reach lengths of 4 to 6 meters and are composed of hundreds of leaflets that sway with the breeze, creating the soothing sound so familiar in tropical environments.

The tree begins flowering at about 6 to 10 years of age, producing both male and female flowers on the same inflorescence. These flowers eventually give rise to the fruit — the coconut — which matures within 11 to 12 months. Each tree can yield between 30 and 100 coconuts annually, depending on variety and growing conditions.

1.3 Varieties and Diversity

THOUGH ALL COCONUTS share a common species name, Cocos nucifera, there are several varieties that differ in size, shape, color, and fruit characteristics. Botanically, coconuts are generally classified into two main groups:

Tall Varieties (Cocos nucifera var. typica): These trees can grow up to 30 meters and live for several decades. They are cross-pollinated, hardy, and produce larger nuts. Examples include the West African Tall and the East Coast Tall.

Dwarf Varieties (Cocos nucifera var. nana): Shorter and more manageable, these trees bear fruit earlier (in 3–4 years) and are often used for ornamental or hybrid purposes. Their water is typically sweeter and more aromatic.

Modern hybrid coconuts combine the best traits of both — the yield and sweetness of dwarfs with the resilience of tall varieties. This hybridization has supported sustainable coconut farming in many tropical countries, helping small farmers increase productivity while preserving biodiversity.

1.4 The Coconut's Ecological Role

BEYOND ITS HUMAN USES, the coconut tree plays an essential role in its natural habitat. Its extensive roots help prevent soil erosion, especially in coastal areas prone to storms and flooding. The fallen leaves and husks decompose into rich organic matter, improving soil fertility and supporting nearby plant growth. Its flowers provide nectar for bees, contributing to pollination and biodiversity.

The tree also supports human livelihoods in ways that promote environmental balance. Coconut farming requires minimal chemical inputs, making it one of the most sustainable crops on earth. The entire plant is biodegradable — a perfect example of a zero-waste system. From an ecological perspective, the coconut embodies what sustainable development should look like: productivity in harmony with nature.

1.5 The Coconut and Humanity: A Historical Partnership

HUMAN HISTORY IS INSEPARABLE from the coconut's story. Ancient explorers and traders carried coconuts across seas as both food and water supply for long voyages. The coconut's shell, husk, and oil were used in household crafts, medicine, and cooking. Early Ayurvedic and African herbal systems recognized it as a universal healer — a remedy for ailments ranging from digestive problems to skin infections.

In the Pacific Islands, the coconut tree was revered as sacred. A well-known Polynesian proverb states, "He who plants a coconut tree plants food, drink, clothing, and shelter for his children." In West Africa, the coconut became a symbol of purity and blessings, often used in traditional rituals, marriages, and festivals.

Even in the modern world, the coconut continues to inspire innovation — from health supplements and cosmetics to biofuel and eco-friendly household products. Its capacity to adapt to human needs is as impressive as its ability to thrive in diverse environments.

1.6 The Science of Survival

ONE OF THE COCONUT'S most extraordinary features is its fruit's design for natural survival and dispersal. The hard shell protects the seed inside, while the fibrous husk allows it to float across seas. Inside, the nutrient-rich water sustains the embryo until it reaches a new shore. When the seed lands, the outer husk gradually decays, forming a natural fertilizer for the sprouting seedling.

This perfect combination of protection, nourishment, and mobility makes the coconut one of the most efficient survival systems in the plant kingdom — a reminder of the intricate intelligence of nature.

1.7 Symbolism and Meaning

ACROSS CULTURES AND faiths, the coconut carries deep symbolic meanings:

In Christianity, it represents purity and divine provision — the outer hardness symbolizing human challenges and the inner sweetness representing God's grace.

In Hinduism and Buddhism, it is offered to deities as a symbol of selflessness and surrender.

In African traditional practices, it signifies truth, cleansing, and fertility.

The coconut's ability to endure harsh conditions and still produce nourishment makes it a universal metaphor for resilience, renewal, and spiritual abundance.

1.8 Summary: Nature's Perfect Design

THE COCONUT TREE STANDS as a living example of harmony — between man and environment, body and spirit, science and nature. From its roots deep in the soil to its crown reaching toward the sun, it embodies the perfect balance of function and beauty.

As we proceed to the next chapters, we will explore how every part of this remarkable plant — roots, stem, leaves, flowers, fruit, and even its by-products — contributes to health, healing, and sustainable living.

The journey of discovery begins here, with gratitude for the wisdom of the earth and the miracle of Cocos nucifera.

2: Nutritional and Medicinal Secrets of the Coconut

2.1 Introduction: Nature's Perfect Pharmacy

In every drop of its water, every shred of its flesh, and every ounce of its oil, the coconut carries a complete package of nutrients, energy, and healing compounds. Long before modern laboratories existed, traditional healers understood the coconut's curative powers. They used its various parts as medicine for fever, wounds, digestive problems, and even mental fatigue.

Today, science confirms what ancient wisdom always knew: the coconut is a functional food — one that not only nourishes but also prevents and heals disease. From its root to its crown, each part of the coconut is rich in unique bioactive compounds that support human health.

2.2 Nutritional Composition of the Coconut

COCONUT'S NUTRITIONAL profile varies slightly depending on the part being used — the water, flesh, milk, or oil — but all share a common trait: dense nutrition in natural balance.

Nutrient	Function	Found In
Medium-Chain Fatty Acids (MCTs)	Provide quick energy, support brain function, boost metabolism	Coconut oil, meat
Lauric Acid	Antiviral, antibacterial, antifungal	Oil, milk
Potassium	Regulates blood pressure, supports hydration	Coconut water
Magnesium	Muscle and nerve function, stress reduction	Meat, water
Iron & Copper	Support red blood cell production	Meat, milk
Vitamin C	Strengthens immunity, aids collagen production	Water, young meat
Vitamin E	Antioxidant, skin protection	Oil
B-Complex Vitamins (B1, B3, B5, B6)	Energy production, brain health	Meat, milk
Dietary Fiber	Aids digestion and bowel health	Water, sprout

THIS NUTRIENT DIVERSITY makes the coconut an exceptional source of hydration, energy, and recovery, especially in hot climates where dehydration and mineral loss are common.

2.3 The Healing Chemistry of the Coconut

A. LAURIC ACID AND Monolaurin

The standout compound in coconut oil is lauric acid, which makes up nearly 50% of its fatty acids. Inside the body, lauric acid is converted to monolaurin, a compound known to destroy lipid-coated viruses such as influenza, herpes, and HIV, as well as bacteria

2.1 Introduction: Nature's Perfect Pharmacy

IN THE GENTLE RUSTLE of its leaves and the cool taste of its water, the coconut tree holds a secret that humanity has only recently begun to rediscover — it is, quite literally, nature's perfect pharmacy. Every part of this extraordinary plant, from its roots beneath the soil to the fruits that hang high above, contains the building blocks of life: nourishment, protection, and healing. For centuries, traditional healers in tropical regions have relied on the coconut not merely as food, but as medicine — a living source of vitality that could restore balance to the human body.

Before science began to isolate nutrients and synthesize drugs, the coconut had already been a trusted companion in natural medicine. It was used to soothe fevers, heal wounds, strengthen the body after illness, and replenish lost energy during long journeys under the tropical sun. The water was valued as a cooling tonic and antidote for dehydration; the flesh served as both food and remedy; and the oil was prized for its cleansing and protective powers. In many ancient healing systems — Ayurvedic, African, Pacific Islander, and Filipino — the coconut was not a luxury, but a daily necessity for wellness.

Modern nutritional science now confirms that these traditions were not based on myth but on chemistry. The coconut is rich in essential fatty acids, vitamins, minerals, and antioxidants that sustain the body's internal balance. It provides clean energy through its unique fats, strengthens immunity through its antimicrobial compounds, and nourishes the brain through its medium-chain triglycerides. What once was passed down through oral wisdom now finds explanation in biochemistry.

Yet the magic of the coconut extends beyond nutrition. It is a living symbol of wholeness — its water representing purity, its meat symbolizing strength, and its oil embodying healing. To study the coconut is to see the marriage between science and spirit, where every molecule tells a story of design and purpose.

In this chapter, we explore the hidden treasures within the coconut: its nutritional composition, its medicinal chemistry, and the scientific foundations that make it one of the most valuable plants in the world. From sustaining the body to protecting against disease, the coconut remains a timeless reminder that nature provides everything we need to live, heal, and thrive.

2.2 Nutritional Composition of the Coconut

THE COCONUT IS OFTEN called the "tree of life" — and rightly so, for within its fruit lies a complete balance of nutrients that sustain both the body and mind. What makes the coconut unique among tropical plants is its ability to offer energy, hydration, fat, and protein in one natural package. From the tender young nut to the mature brown shell, every stage of its growth provides a distinct nutritional profile and purpose.

At its core, the coconut fruit is divided into three edible components: the water, the meat, and the oil. Coconut water, found in young green coconuts, is nature's most pristine beverage. It is composed of 95% water, enriched with electrolytes such as potassium, sodium, magnesium, and calcium. These minerals make it an ideal natural rehydration fluid, comparable in composition to human plasma. It restores lost fluids during illness or physical exertion and maintains the body's electrolyte balance, which is vital for nerve and muscle function. In emergency cases, coconut water has even been used as an intravenous hydration fluid during wartime, a testament to its purity and compatibility with the human body.

The flesh, or coconut meat, contains a higher concentration of nutrients. It provides dietary fiber, protein, and healthy fats — particularly medium-chain triglycerides (MCTs), which the body metabolizes quickly for energy rather than storing as fat. These fats also have antimicrobial properties, helping to combat harmful bacteria, viruses, and fungi. Additionally, the meat contains essential vitamins such as C, E, B1, B3, B5, and B6, along with minerals like iron, selenium, phosphorus, and zinc. Together, these nutrients nourish cells, support metabolism, and enhance immune function.

Coconut oil, extracted from the dried flesh known as copra, is one of the richest natural sources of lauric acid, a compound that strengthens immunity and promotes cardiovascular health. Lauric acid converts into monolaurin in the body, a substance known for destroying lipid-coated viruses and pathogens. The oil's unique molecular structure also makes it an excellent energy source for the brain, which is why it has become popular in modern nutrition as a natural aid for cognitive health and memory enhancement.

Beyond the fruit, even the outer husk and shell hold nutritional and medicinal relevance. The shell charcoal is used to purify water and detoxify the body, while extracts from the husk have been studied for their antioxidant and antimicrobial effects. Every layer of the coconut seems designed for life — from the cooling liquid within to the protective shell that guards it.

In essence, the coconut's nutritional composition mirrors the completeness of nature itself. It provides hydration, sustenance, and healing in perfect balance — a living demonstration that true nourishment comes not from artificial mixtures, but from the intelligent design of creation.

2.3 Medicinal Compounds and Their Healing Mechanisms

THE COCONUT IS MORE than a source of food; it is a natural pharmacy packed with bioactive compounds that nurture, protect, and restore the human body. The healing properties long recognized in traditional medicine now find validation in scientific studies that explore its antimicrobial, antiviral, anti-inflammatory, and antioxidant characteristics. Each component of the coconut contributes to health through a unique interplay of natural chemicals that operate at the cellular and systemic levels.

One of the most remarkable compounds found in the coconut is lauric acid, which makes up nearly half of the fatty acids in coconut oil. When consumed, lauric acid is converted into monolaurin — a substance known for its ability to destroy lipid-coated viruses such as HIV, influenza, herpes, and measles. Monolaurin works by dissolving the protective lipid membrane surrounding these pathogens, rendering them inactive and vulnerable to the immune system's defenses. This same mechanism also helps to control harmful bacteria and fungi in the digestive tract, promoting a healthier gut microbiome and enhancing nutrient absorption.

Coconut oil also contains caprylic acid, capric acid, and myristic acid, which work synergistically with lauric acid to inhibit microbial growth and reduce inflammation. These medium-chain fatty acids not only act as natural antibiotics but also serve as quick energy sources for the liver and brain. Unlike long-chain fats that are stored in the body, these medium-chain triglycerides (MCTs) are rapidly metabolized, helping to improve metabolism, support weight balance, and stabilize blood sugar levels.

Beyond the fats, the coconut's polyphenols and antioxidants play a crucial role in protecting cells from oxidative stress. Compounds such as catechins, ferulic acid, and p-coumaric acid help neutralize free radicals — unstable molecules that contribute to aging and chronic diseases. By reducing oxidative damage, these antioxidants enhance cardiovascular health, protect neural tissues, and promote youthful skin. They also support liver detoxification and may reduce the risk of cancer by preventing DNA damage.

The coconut's medicinal potential extends to its water as well. Rich in cytokinins, a group of plant hormones, coconut water exhibits anti-aging and anti-carcinogenic properties. Cytokinins help regulate cell growth and repair, ensuring that tissues remain healthy and resilient. In traditional practices, coconut water has been used to treat urinary tract infections, kidney stones, and dehydration-related disorders due to its diuretic and cleansing properties.

The fiber in coconut meat further enhances these healing effects by supporting digestive health. It helps regulate bowel movement, bind toxins, and maintain a balanced gut ecosystem. When combined with the antimicrobial fats and antioxidants, the coconut forms a complete therapeutic system — cleansing, nourishing, and protecting from within.

Thus, the coconut's healing power lies not in a single compound but in its synergy — a natural harmony where each element amplifies the effect of the other. It acts gently yet profoundly, restoring the body's equilibrium without disturbing its natural rhythms. This balance between nourishment and medicine makes the coconut a true emblem of holistic health.

2.4 Coconut in Traditional and Modern Medicine

ACROSS CONTINENTS AND centuries, the coconut has been revered not just as a source of sustenance but as a divine gift of healing. In traditional societies, healers recognized the coconut's diverse uses long before laboratories confirmed its medicinal properties. Its symbolism of purity, renewal, and vitality found expression in both cultural rituals and medical practices — an enduring testament to its role as a natural healer.

In Ayurvedic medicine, practiced in India for over three thousand years, the coconut is classified as sattvic — pure, cooling, and life-sustaining. It is said to balance the pitta dosha, calming internal heat and inflammation. Ayurvedic physicians recommend coconut water for reducing fever, improving digestion, and soothing urinary tract infections. The oil, when applied to the scalp and body, is believed to nourish the tissues (dhatus), strengthen the nervous system, and purify the skin. It is also used in oil-pulling, an ancient oral detoxification method that removes toxins, strengthens the gums, and refreshes the mouth.

In the Pacific Islands, where the coconut tree is called the tree of life, its parts are used to treat nearly every ailment known to the local people. The roots are boiled to make tea for diarrhea and dysentery; the sap from the flower bud is fermented into a drink believed to enhance vitality; and the oil is applied to wounds, burns, and infections to promote rapid healing. The elders often refer to coconut oil as a "living salve," combining nourishment and protection in one simple remedy.

Among African traditional healers, especially in West and Central Africa, the coconut is used in both physical and spiritual healing. Coconut oil is rubbed on the chest to relieve coughs and bronchitis, or mixed with herbs to treat skin infections and rashes. In many communities, the coconut also carries spiritual significance — symbolizing truth, purity, and new beginnings. During healing rituals, the breaking of a coconut often represents the release of negativity and the restoration of health.

Modern medicine, guided by scientific inquiry, has begun to validate these age-old practices. Research confirms that virgin coconut oil possesses antimicrobial, antifungal, and antiviral properties, supporting immune defense and skin health. Studies on MCTs (medium-chain triglycerides) show improvements in cognitive function, particularly in Alzheimer's patients, by providing an alternative fuel source to glucose for the brain. Furthermore, coconut water has been shown to aid recovery from dehydration, support cardiovascular health, and even lower blood pressure due to its potassium content.

The convergence of traditional and modern perspectives on the coconut underscores a profound truth: that ancient wisdom often precedes scientific discovery. The coconut bridges this gap, uniting the holistic insights of ancestral healers with the empirical methods of contemporary science. As medicine continues to evolve toward integrative and natural approaches, the coconut remains a shining example of harmony between tradition and innovation.

In essence, whether offered at a shrine, prescribed in an herbal concoction, or bottled in a modern health store, the coconut continues to affirm its timeless role as nature's physician — accessible, balanced, and deeply healing.

2.5 Scientific Evidence Supporting Coconut's Health Benefits

WHILE TRADITIONAL MEDICINE laid the foundation for the therapeutic use of coconut, scientific research has built upon that knowledge with precision and evidence. In recent decades, laboratories around the world have examined the biochemical properties of the coconut to understand why it works as effectively as folk healers have claimed. The results have been remarkable, revealing that the coconut's healing power is rooted in measurable physiological and molecular mechanisms.

One of the most extensively studied components is coconut oil, particularly virgin coconut oil (VCO). Clinical and laboratory studies have confirmed that VCO possesses significant antimicrobial and antiviral activity. Research published in the Journal of Medicinal Food (2009) demonstrated that monolaurin, derived from lauric acid, inactivates lipid-coated viruses such as influenza, HIV, and herpes simplex by dissolving their protective membranes. This same compound also inhibits Candida albicans, a common fungal pathogen responsible for yeast infections, by disrupting its cell membrane integrity.

Studies have further shown that consuming moderate amounts of coconut oil can enhance metabolism and fat oxidation. A study in the American Journal of Clinical Nutrition (2015) found that medium-chain triglycerides (MCTs) increase energy expenditure compared to long-chain fats, making them useful in weight management and obesity prevention. The liver rapidly converts MCTs into ketones — an alternative fuel source for the brain — which has led to the use of coconut oil in neurodegenerative conditions such as Alzheimer's disease. Research from the Journal of Alzheimer's Disease (2017) reported improved cognitive performance in patients who incorporated MCTs into their diet.

Coconut's antioxidant and anti-inflammatory effects have also been well documented. Scientists at the University of Kerala (India) found that virgin coconut oil increased antioxidant enzyme activity and reduced oxidative stress in laboratory animals. These effects are attributed to phenolic compounds such as ferulic acid, catechins, and p-coumaric acid, which protect cells from free radical damage. Such protection contributes to cardiovascular health by reducing lipid peroxidation and maintaining healthy cholesterol levels — increasing HDL (good cholesterol) while lowering LDL (bad cholesterol).

Coconut water, once considered merely a refreshing drink, has now gained recognition as a natural electrolyte solution and a mild diuretic.

Studies published in Food and Function (2018) confirm its efficacy in restoring hydration and maintaining electrolyte balance after strenuous exercise or illness. Its potassium and magnesium content support heart function, while cytokinins in the water show anti-aging effects by regulating cell division and delaying senescence in tissues.

Moreover, the fibrous components of coconut meat play a role in digestive health. According to research in the Journal of Functional Foods (2016), coconut dietary fiber promotes beneficial gut bacteria, reduces cholesterol absorption, and prevents constipation. These fibers act synergistically with the oil's antimicrobial properties, enhancing overall gut integrity and immunity.

The cosmetic and dermatological applications of coconut have also received scientific backing. A study in Dermatitis (2008) revealed that virgin coconut oil is as effective as mineral oil in moisturizing skin, but with additional antibacterial and anti-inflammatory effects. It is particularly beneficial for conditions such as eczema and dermatitis due to its ability to reduce bacterial colonization and restore the skin barrier.

Altogether, these findings affirm that the coconut's health benefits are not coincidental but are deeply rooted in biochemistry. Its components — fats, polyphenols, minerals, and phytonutrients — work in a coordinated manner to nourish, protect, and heal. The scientific validation of traditional wisdom underscores an enduring truth: nature's medicines are complete in themselves, awaiting only our willingness to understand and use them wisely.

2.6 The Holistic Philosophy Behind Coconut Healing

THE THERAPEUTIC POTENTIAL of the coconut cannot be fully understood through biochemical analysis alone. While modern science has effectively quantified its nutritional and pharmacological value, the deeper significance of the coconut lies in its representation of holistic health — a philosophy that perceives the human body, mind, and environment as an integrated system. Within this paradigm, the coconut functions not merely as a source of nutrients but as a medium for restoring balance and harmony between physiological processes and natural forces.

The holistic perspective is grounded in the belief that health is not the absence of disease but the presence of equilibrium. In this sense, the coconut embodies a synergistic system of healing, in which each of its components—water, meat, oil, husk, and root—contributes to maintaining internal stability. Its biochemical compounds act on multiple levels: the physical (through nourishment and protection), the biochemical (through immune and metabolic modulation), and the energetic (through cleansing and cooling properties). This multidimensionality aligns closely with traditional systems such as Ayurveda and naturopathy, where treatment focuses on supporting the body's innate capacity to heal rather than suppressing symptoms.

In the Ayurvedic framework, the coconut is regarded as tridoshic—capable of balancing all three doshas (vata, pitta, and kapha) when used appropriately. Its cooling nature mitigates internal heat and inflammation, while its nourishing oils strengthen tissues and the nervous system. The oil's application to the scalp and skin symbolizes restoration not only of the body's moisture but also of mental calmness and clarity. Thus, coconut healing extends beyond physical repair; it fosters psychological and emotional stability, key determinants of holistic well-being.

From an ecological and philosophical standpoint, the coconut also exemplifies sustainability in healing. Each part of the plant serves a purpose, ensuring that nothing is wasted. This mirrors the holistic view that wellness must include environmental consciousness — the understanding that human health is inseparable from the health of the natural world. The coconut's ability to thrive in saline soils and harsh coastal conditions further symbolizes resilience, adaptability, and the regenerative principles of life itself.

Contemporary holistic medicine increasingly recognizes the importance of such integrative paradigms. Researchers in integrative nutrition and functional medicine argue that isolated nutrients, when extracted from their natural context, lose part of their therapeutic potential. The coconut's efficacy arises from its complex composition and the synergy among its constituents, which act together to produce comprehensive healing effects. This synergy cannot be replicated in synthetic formulations, reaffirming the superiority of whole-food-based interventions in preventive and restorative health care.

In conclusion, the holistic philosophy surrounding coconut healing underscores a vital academic insight: health cannot be understood or achieved through reductionism alone. It requires the integration of empirical science, traditional wisdom, and ecological ethics. The coconut, as a model of this integration, invites scholars and practitioners to adopt a more systemic approach to nutrition and medicine—one that values the harmony between human biology and the natural environment.

3: Healing from the Roots

3.1 The Coconut Roots: Detoxification and Medicinal Uses

The roots of the coconut tree, often overlooked in contemporary health discourse, constitute one of the most potent yet underutilized parts of the plant. Traditionally employed in indigenous and rural medicine across Asia, Africa, and the Pacific Islands, coconut roots have been valued for their cleansing, detoxifying, and restorative properties. From a scientific and ethnobotanical perspective, these roots represent a phytochemical reservoir that contributes significantly to the coconut's holistic medicinal system.

Chemically, coconut roots contain a range of bioactive compounds including tannins, saponins, flavonoids, and phenolic acids. These compounds exhibit antioxidant, antimicrobial, and anti-inflammatory activities, thereby supporting the body's detoxification processes. Tannins act as natural astringents, tightening tissues and reducing inflammation in the gastrointestinal tract, while saponins facilitate the removal of metabolic wastes by enhancing kidney and liver function. Flavonoids, meanwhile, neutralize free radicals and improve blood circulation, thereby strengthening the body's overall resilience against oxidative stress.

In traditional medicine, decoctions made from the roots are administered as diuretics and blood purifiers. In Ayurvedic and Pacific Island practices, boiled coconut roots are used to treat urinary tract infections, diarrhea, dysentery, and fever. The diuretic effect assists in flushing toxins through increased urine output, while the antimicrobial properties help to eliminate pathogens from the urinary and digestive systems. In African herbal traditions, the same root infusions are consumed to cleanse the blood, manage menstrual irregularities, and reduce joint inflammation associated with rheumatism or gout.

Empirical studies have begun to validate these traditional uses. Research published in the Journal of Ethnopharmacology (2013) confirmed that methanolic extracts of coconut roots demonstrated significant antimicrobial activity against Escherichia coli, Staphylococcus aureus, and Candida albicans. Additional analyses revealed the presence of secondary metabolites with potential hepatoprotective effects, suggesting that coconut root extracts could aid in liver detoxification and the prevention of toxin-induced hepatic damage.

Beyond internal detoxification, coconut roots are also used externally in traditional healing. Root paste or decoction, when applied to wounds, accelerates healing through its astringent and antiseptic properties. The fibrous root system, when charred and powdered, is occasionally used as a natural dental cleaning agent, helping to remove plaque and strengthen the gums—an ancient practice still observed in some rural communities.

Philosophically, the coconut root symbolizes the grounding principle in holistic healing—the idea that wellness begins from the foundation. Just as roots anchor and nourish the tree, human health depends on the integrity of internal cleansing systems such as the liver, kidneys, and colon. The coconut root, therefore, functions as both a literal and metaphorical agent of purification, linking physiological detoxification with the broader concept of renewal and balance.

In summary, the coconut root offers a unique intersection of tradition and modern science. Its biochemical richness and therapeutic versatility position it as an important natural detoxifier within integrative health systems. Future pharmacological studies hold promise for uncovering new applications of these roots, particularly in the management of metabolic and inflammatory disorders. The inclusion of coconut root therapies in holistic medicine may thus contribute to more sustainable, plant-based approaches to detoxification and overall well-being.

3.2 Preparation and Applications of Coconut Root Remedies

THE MEDICINAL POTENCY of coconut roots is best realized when they are carefully prepared and administered according to traditional or scientifically informed methods. Preparation determines the extraction efficiency of the bioactive compounds contained within the roots, and thus influences the overall therapeutic effect. The following discussion presents key preparation approaches and their corresponding applications, integrating traditional wisdom with modern pharmacognostic understanding.

The most common preparation is the root decoction, which involves boiling fresh or dried coconut roots in clean water for approximately twenty to thirty minutes. This process extracts the water-soluble tannins, saponins, and flavonoids that are responsible for the detoxifying and antimicrobial effects. The resulting brownish liquid is typically consumed warm, one to two times daily, to treat ailments such as urinary infections, digestive disturbances, and general body fatigue. In some traditions, honey or palm sugar is added to the decoction to enhance palatability and provide additional energy to the convalescing patient.

For liver detoxification and blood purification, the decoction is often combined with small amounts of lime juice or turmeric powder. The acidity of the lime enhances absorption, while the curcuminoids in turmeric amplify the anti-inflammatory response. This combination illustrates the integrative principle in traditional medicine—where synergy among natural ingredients magnifies the therapeutic potential of each component. Empirical observation suggests that consistent use of this preparation supports clearer skin, improved digestion, and a general sense of lightness associated with reduced toxic load.

Another widely utilized form is the root infusion, a milder preparation obtained by steeping chopped roots in hot water without boiling. This method preserves heat-sensitive antioxidants and is recommended for daily consumption as a preventive tonic. Herbalists prescribe this infusion to improve kidney function, regulate blood pressure, and support the body's natural cleansing cycles. It also acts as a gentle diuretic, assisting in the removal of metabolic wastes while maintaining electrolyte balance.

The external applications of coconut root preparations are equally valuable. A paste made from ground roots mixed with coconut oil or aloe vera gel can be applied to skin infections, boils, and wounds to reduce microbial load and inflammation. The combination of root extracts and coconut oil provides both antiseptic and moisturizing properties, facilitating tissue repair without leaving scars. In certain rural settings, this same preparation is used as a foot soak to alleviate swelling, fungal infections, and fatigue caused by prolonged walking or labor.

A lesser-known but culturally significant practice involves using charred coconut roots as a form of natural charcoal. When powdered and mixed with salt, this preparation serves as an effective dental cleanser that helps eliminate bacteria and strengthen the gums. Its mild abrasive quality removes plaque, while the antibacterial action reduces oral infections. Such traditional practices, now being re-evaluated by modern herbal dentistry, reflect the sustainable use of every part of the coconut plant in maintaining health and hygiene.

Phytochemical investigations suggest that the efficacy of these preparations depends largely on the concentration and stability of active compounds. Therefore, for modern application, standardized extraction methods and dosage guidelines are essential to ensure safety and reproducibility. Future pharmaceutical development could focus on encapsulating or formulating coconut root extracts into teas, tinctures, or supplements, thus bridging traditional knowledge with contemporary therapeutic standards.

In conclusion, coconut root remedies exemplify the harmony between empirical tradition and scientific inquiry. Whether used as simple household decoctions or as candidates for modern herbal formulations, they represent a valuable, sustainable, and culturally embedded resource for natural health care. Their continued exploration promises to deepen our understanding of plant-based detoxification and the enduring wisdom of indigenous healing systems.

3.3 Scientific Studies on Coconut Root Phytochemistry

SCIENTIFIC INTEREST in the phytochemical profile of coconut roots has increased over the past two decades, as researchers seek to validate and expand upon the therapeutic claims rooted in traditional medicine. Phytochemistry, the study of bioactive compounds in plants, provides the scientific framework for understanding how these natural constituents exert their physiological and pharmacological effects. In the case of the coconut tree (Cocos nucifera L.), studies have revealed that the roots are a rich source of diverse secondary metabolites that possess antioxidant, antimicrobial, anti-inflammatory, and hepatoprotective properties.

Analytical studies using techniques such as gas chromatography-mass spectrometry (GC-MS), high-performance liquid chromatography

(HPLC), and spectrophotometry have identified numerous phytoconstituents in coconut root extracts. The primary groups include flavonoids, tannins, saponins, alkaloids, terpenoids, and phenolic acids. Each of these classes contributes uniquely to the plant's medicinal efficacy. Flavonoids, for instance, are known for their capacity to scavenge free radicals and regulate enzymatic activity involved in oxidative stress. Tannins serve as potent astringents and antimicrobial agents, while saponins enhance cellular permeability and contribute to detoxification processes.

A study conducted by Suresh et al. (2013) in the Journal of Ethnopharmacology examined the methanolic extract of Cocos nucifera roots and found significant antimicrobial activity against Staphylococcus aureus, Escherichia coli, and Candida albicans. The same study demonstrated notable antioxidant activity, indicating that the extract could play a role in preventing oxidative damage at the cellular level. Another investigation by Rahman and colleagues (2016) revealed that aqueous root extracts exhibited hepatoprotective effects in laboratory rats subjected to carbon tetrachloride-induced liver toxicity. The treated animals showed marked improvement in liver enzyme levels, suggesting that coconut root constituents support hepatic regeneration and function.

In a more recent comparative analysis (Singh et al., 2021), researchers evaluated the phytochemical composition of coconut roots grown in different soil conditions. They observed variations in phenolic content and antioxidant capacity, indicating that environmental factors significantly influence the bioactive profile of the roots. This finding underscores the importance of ecological considerations in the cultivation and standardization of medicinal plants. The study also identified specific phenolic acids—such as gallic acid, caffeic acid, and ferulic acid—which have been associated with anti-inflammatory and anticancer activities in other plant systems.

Additionally, preliminary pharmacokinetic modeling has suggested that several compounds present in coconut roots exhibit favorable absorption and bioavailability characteristics, making them viable candidates for therapeutic development. For instance, saponin derivatives extracted from the roots have been shown to possess surface-active properties that could enhance the delivery of other bioactive molecules within the human body. This finding aligns with the broader pharmacognostic interest in plant-based compounds that can serve as natural drug carriers or synergistic agents in multi-component therapies.

Toxicological assessments, though limited, have thus far indicated that coconut root extracts are safe for consumption at traditional dosages. However, higher concentrations may cause mild gastrointestinal discomfort, emphasizing the need for standardized dosing in future clinical applications. The absence of acute toxicity supports the traditional view of coconut roots as gentle yet effective detoxifiers—a profile consistent with other medicinal roots such as ginger and turmeric.

Collectively, these scientific studies validate many of the empirical uses of coconut roots and open pathways for further exploration. The intersection of phytochemistry and pharmacology reveals the complexity and potential of this often-overlooked part of the coconut tree. Continued investigation into its molecular mechanisms, synergistic interactions, and therapeutic applications could lead to the development of novel plant-based interventions for metabolic, hepatic, and infectious diseases. In this respect, the coconut root stands as both an ancient remedy and a modern subject of biomedical relevance.

3.4 DIY Coconut Root Tonics and Herbal Preparations

THE PRACTICAL APPLICATION of coconut root in daily health routines can be realized through carefully prepared tonics and herbal remedies. Drawing from both traditional practices and contemporary understanding of phytochemistry, these preparations maximize the bioavailability of active compounds while ensuring safety and efficacy. For students, health enthusiasts, and practitioners, creating such formulations at home provides a tangible way to integrate coconut root therapy into holistic wellness strategies.

Root Decoction for Internal Detoxification

The most accessible and widely used preparation is a decoction derived from fresh or dried coconut roots. Begin by cleaning the roots thoroughly to remove soil and debris. Chop them into small pieces and boil in approximately two liters of water for twenty to thirty minutes, or until the water reduces by half. Strain the liquid to remove solid particles. This decoction can be consumed warm or at room temperature, one cup in the morning and one in the evening. Its primary applications include promoting kidney and liver function, supporting urinary health, and acting as a general detoxifying agent.

Infusion for Gentle Daily Tonic

For a milder preparation, a root infusion can be employed. Steep cleaned and chopped roots in hot water without boiling for ten to fifteen minutes. This method preserves heat-sensitive antioxidants and provides a gentle tonic suitable for daily consumption. Regular use is believed to enhance metabolic efficiency, improve digestion, and sustain immune resilience.

External Applications for Skin and Wound Care

Coconut root can also be formulated into pastes or poultices for topical use. Grind the roots into a fine powder and combine with a carrier medium such as virgin coconut oil or aloe vera gel to create a smooth paste. Apply directly to minor cuts, abrasions, boils, or inflammatory skin conditions. The astringent, antimicrobial, and anti-inflammatory properties of the root extract facilitate tissue repair, reduce microbial load, and promote localized healing. In some practices, the paste is applied to swollen joints or sore muscles to alleviate discomfort and improve circulation.

Dental and Oral Health Preparations

Charred coconut roots, when powdered and combined with salt or baking soda, serve as an effective natural dental cleanser. Brushing gently with this mixture helps remove plaque, reduce bacterial colonization, and strengthen the gums. The combination of mild abrasives and antimicrobial compounds provides an eco-friendly alternative to commercial oral care products.

Synergistic Herbal Formulations

In traditional herbalism, coconut root is often combined with complementary plant materials to enhance efficacy. For instance, adding turmeric to the decoction increases anti-inflammatory effects, while the inclusion of lime juice or honey improves both palatability and therapeutic potential. Such formulations illustrate the principle of synergy in phytotherapy: multiple natural compounds working together can provide broader and more balanced health benefits than any single ingredient in isolation.

Safety Considerations

Although coconut root preparations are generally safe when consumed in traditional quantities, caution should be exercised with higher concentrations, particularly in individuals with sensitive gastrointestinal systems. Pregnant and lactating women should consult healthcare providers before incorporating root tonics, and all preparations should be made using clean, uncontaminated water to prevent microbial contamination.

In summary, DIY coconut root tonics and herbal preparations bridge traditional knowledge and modern practice, offering practical methods to harness the plant's detoxifying and restorative properties. By adhering to careful preparation techniques and informed application, individuals can integrate the roots of the coconut tree into their daily health regimen, promoting systemic balance, resilience, and holistic well-being.

3.5 Recipes Incorporating Coconut Root for Culinary and Therapeutic Use

WHILE COCONUT ROOTS are primarily recognized for their medicinal applications, they can also be thoughtfully incorporated into culinary practices, creating preparations that serve both nutritional and therapeutic purposes. Integrating coconut root into recipes provides an avenue to enhance systemic health while maintaining the sensory and cultural dimensions of food. Below are carefully developed examples that balance efficacy, palatability, and simplicity.

Coconut Root Herbal Broth

This preparation serves as a nourishing tonic suitable for individuals recovering from illness or experiencing fatigue. Begin by cleaning and slicing 100–150 grams of fresh coconut root. Boil the roots in 1.5 liters of water for 25–30 minutes, then add a small portion of sliced ginger and a pinch of turmeric powder. Reduce the liquid to approximately one liter. The resulting broth can be consumed warm, one cup in the morning and one in the evening. The combination of coconut root, ginger, and turmeric provides synergistic anti-inflammatory, antioxidant, and digestive-supportive effects, making it ideal for internal detoxification and immune reinforcement.

Coconut Root Infused Tea

A lighter preparation suitable for daily consumption involves steeping 50 grams of cleaned, chopped coconut root in hot water for 10–15 minutes. Sweeten minimally with honey or a natural sugar alternative. This tea acts as a gentle diuretic, supporting kidney function, and is recommended for maintaining electrolyte balance during periods of mild dehydration or physical exertion.

Coconut Root and Vegetable Soup

For a more substantive dish, coconut root can be incorporated into soups and stews. Peel and chop 100 grams of coconut root into thin slices and add to a simmering mixture of local vegetables such as spinach, carrots, and pumpkin. Season lightly with salt, herbs, and a small quantity of coconut oil to enhance flavor and nutritional value. Simmer for 20–25 minutes until the root softens. This preparation provides dietary fiber, micronutrients, and phytochemicals while retaining the therapeutic properties of the coconut root.

Topical Coconut Root Paste for Culinary and Medicinal Use

Although not ingested, the root can be integrated into topical applications that complement dietary use. Grind coconut roots into a fine powder and blend with virgin coconut oil to create a paste that can be applied to minor skin irritations or as part of a wellness ritual. Incorporating fresh herbs such as aloe vera or neem enhances both antimicrobial and anti-inflammatory efficacy.

Coconut Root Smoothie Adaptation

For contemporary culinary applications, a powdered or finely grated form of coconut root can be added to smoothies. Combine 10–15 grams of powdered root with coconut water, banana, and a small amount of honey. The smoothie provides hydration, essential electrolytes, and gentle detoxifying compounds, offering a functional beverage that merges taste with health-promoting properties.

In crafting these recipes, attention must be paid to preparation methods that preserve the active compounds. Excessive boiling or high-heat exposure may reduce the concentration of certain antioxidants and heat-sensitive phytochemicals. Therefore, moderate temperatures and minimal cooking times are recommended for maximizing therapeutic benefit.

Collectively, these culinary approaches exemplify how coconut root can be seamlessly incorporated into daily life. They reinforce the concept that food and medicine need not be distinct; instead, thoughtful integration of phytochemically rich ingredients such as coconut root can simultaneously satisfy nutritional requirements and support systemic health.

4: The Stem and Its Hidden Health Power

4.1 Coconut Trunk and Bark: Health and Practical Applications

The coconut trunk and bark, often overlooked in the study of the plant's medicinal and practical uses, possess a range of properties that contribute to both human health and sustainable living. While the trunk primarily serves structural and industrial purposes, the bark contains bioactive compounds that have been recognized in ethnomedicine and emerging scientific research. Understanding these components expands the conceptual framework of the coconut as a holistic resource.

From an ethnopharmacological perspective, the bark of the coconut tree has been used in traditional medicine to address inflammatory conditions, gastrointestinal disturbances, and infections. Decoctions made from dried bark are consumed as tonics to reduce fever, alleviate diarrhea, and support detoxification. The bark contains phenolic compounds, tannins, and lignans, which exhibit antimicrobial, astringent, and antioxidant activities. Tannins, in particular, contribute to the reduction of intestinal inflammation and the mitigation of microbial overgrowth in the digestive tract. In rural communities, bark infusions have been utilized as mild antiseptics, applied to external wounds and skin irritations to prevent infection and promote healing.

The coconut trunk, while less commonly ingested, also holds practical medicinal value. Young, sap-rich sections of the trunk, often called toddy wood, are used in some cultures for their cooling and hydrating properties. The sap extracted from incisions in the trunk contains sugars, electrolytes, and trace minerals that serve as a natural energy source and mild tonic. Fermented sap has been employed traditionally to manage gastrointestinal discomfort and support general vitality.

Beyond internal medicinal uses, the trunk and bark play a significant role in topical and external applications. Charred or powdered bark is sometimes incorporated into poultices or ointments to treat minor skin abrasions, insect bites, or localized inflammation. The combination of phenolics and tannins in the bark contributes to its antibacterial and anti-inflammatory effects, facilitating wound healing. In addition, fiber extracted from the inner trunk has historically been used to create mats, ropes, and padding, demonstrating the multifunctionality of the coconut in both health and daily life.

Modern scientific studies have begun to explore these traditional claims. In vitro experiments demonstrate that extracts from coconut bark exhibit measurable antibacterial activity against pathogens such as Staphylococcus aureus and Escherichia coli. Antioxidant assays further indicate that phenolic-rich bark extracts can neutralize free radicals, suggesting potential applications in managing oxidative stress and inflammatory disorders. These findings lend empirical support to centuries of indigenous knowledge, reinforcing the coconut's status as a multi-component medicinal resource.

From a holistic perspective, the utilization of trunk and bark emphasizes the principle of zero-waste medicine, in which each part of a plant contributes to human health or practical utility. While much attention has historically focused on the fruit, oil, and roots, the trunk and bark exemplify the comprehensive nature of the coconut tree as a therapeutic and functional organism. Their integration into health practices not only provides medicinal benefits but also encourages sustainable and resource-efficient approaches to herbal medicine.

In summary, the coconut trunk and bark, though less prominent in culinary or direct nutritional applications, offer substantive contributions to ethnomedicine and practical wellness. Their bioactive compounds, coupled with traditional methods of preparation, provide anti-inflammatory, antimicrobial, and detoxifying benefits. Recognizing these uses expands the holistic understanding of the coconut tree and reinforces its value as a comprehensive, multifunctional natural resource.

4.2 Preparation and Application of Coconut Trunk and Bark Remedies

THE THERAPEUTIC USE of coconut trunk and bark relies on appropriate preparation methods that optimize the extraction and preservation of bioactive compounds. Traditional practices, corroborated by modern phytochemical research, provide guidance on creating remedies that are both effective and safe. This section outlines preparation techniques and practical applications for internal and external use, highlighting the integration of empirical knowledge and contemporary understanding.

Decoctions and Infusions for Internal Use

Coconut bark is commonly prepared as a decoction for systemic health benefits. The bark should first be cleaned thoroughly to remove soil and impurities. Once dried, it can be chopped into small pieces and boiled in water for 20–30 minutes, until the liquid reduces to the desired concentration. The resulting decoction can be consumed in small amounts—typically one cup twice daily—to support gastrointestinal health, reduce inflammation, and promote detoxification. For a milder alternative, an infusion can be prepared by steeping the cleaned bark in hot water for 10–15 minutes. This method preserves delicate antioxidants and is suitable for individuals seeking a gentle tonic.

Topical Poultices and Ointments

Coconut bark can also be employed externally for skin conditions and minor injuries. The powdered bark may be mixed with virgin coconut oil or aloe vera gel to form a paste. This preparation can be applied to abrasions, insect bites, or areas of localized inflammation. The phenolic compounds and tannins present in the bark confer antimicrobial and astringent properties, facilitating wound healing and reducing microbial proliferation. For more severe skin infections, the bark paste may be combined with other medicinal herbs, such as turmeric or neem, to enhance anti-inflammatory and antiseptic effects.

Sap-Based Tonics from the Trunk

The young sections of the coconut trunk yield sap, which can be harvested by careful incision of the stem. Fresh sap contains sugars, electrolytes, and trace minerals that provide energy and hydration. It can be consumed directly as a tonic or lightly fermented to create a mildly effervescent beverage that retains its mineral and enzymatic content. This sap is traditionally used to alleviate fatigue, support gastrointestinal function, and promote general vitality.

Charred Bark for Dental and Antiseptic Use

In certain traditional applications, the bark is charred, powdered, and combined with salt or baking soda to create a natural antiseptic powder. This formulation can be used for oral hygiene, aiding in plaque removal and gum strengthening, or applied to minor skin abrasions to prevent infection. The astringent qualities of tannins in the charred bark reinforce tissue contraction and healing.

Synergistic Formulations

Coconut trunk and bark remedies are often enhanced by combining them with other botanicals to maximize therapeutic potential. For example, bark decoctions may include ginger, turmeric, or lemongrass to augment anti-inflammatory, antioxidant, and antimicrobial activity. These synergistic combinations illustrate the principle of phytochemical cooperation, wherein multiple natural compounds interact to produce more comprehensive health effects than individual constituents alone.

Safety and Dosage Considerations

Although coconut trunk and bark preparations are generally considered safe, excessive consumption or improper preparation may cause gastrointestinal discomfort or mild allergic reactions. Decoctions should be prepared with clean water, and topical applications should be tested on a small area of skin to ensure tolerance. Pregnant or lactating individuals should seek medical guidance before using these remedies, and all preparations should follow standardized measurements to optimize efficacy and safety.

In summary, the preparation and application of coconut trunk and bark remedies demonstrate the intersection of traditional herbal knowledge and contemporary phytochemical insight. Properly executed decoctions, infusions, pastes, and sap-based tonics offer significant health benefits, including antimicrobial, anti-inflammatory, and detoxifying effects. These methods underscore the coconut tree's holistic potential, highlighting its role as a multifaceted natural resource capable of promoting systemic well-being through diverse modalities.

4.3 Recipes and DIY Uses of Coconut Trunk and Bark

THE INTEGRATION OF coconut trunk and bark into culinary and household applications demonstrates the versatility of this often-overlooked component of the coconut tree. Beyond traditional medicinal use, these parts can be incorporated into recipes and DIY preparations that support wellness, hygiene, and environmental sustainability. This section outlines practical methods to utilize the trunk and bark, highlighting both therapeutic and functional applications.

Coconut Bark Herbal Tea

A simple and accessible recipe involves preparing coconut bark as a herbal tea. Clean and slice 30–50 grams of dried bark and steep it in 500 milliliters of hot water for 10–15 minutes. Sweeten minimally with honey or a natural sweetener to enhance palatability. This tea provides antioxidants, tannins, and trace minerals, supporting gastrointestinal health, detoxification, and mild anti-inflammatory effects. Regular consumption may assist in maintaining systemic balance and overall wellness.

Coconut Bark and Ginger Decoction

For enhanced digestive and anti-inflammatory benefits, the bark can be combined with ginger. Boil 50 grams of bark and a 20-gram piece of fresh ginger in one liter of water for 20–25 minutes. Strain and consume warm. This preparation is traditionally used to alleviate digestive discomfort, reduce fever, and support metabolic function. The combination of phenolic compounds from the bark and bioactive ginger constituents exemplifies a synergistic approach to herbal therapy.

Topical Bark Paste for Skin Care

Coconut bark can be transformed into a topical remedy by grinding it into a fine powder and mixing with virgin coconut oil to form a smooth paste. Apply the paste to minor skin irritations, rashes, or insect bites to reduce inflammation and microbial activity. For enhanced efficacy, small amounts of turmeric or neem powder may be added. This DIY remedy provides an eco-friendly alternative to commercial antiseptics while leveraging the antimicrobial and astringent properties of the bark.

Sap-Based Beverage from Young Trunk Sections

Sap extracted from young coconut trunk sections can be consumed directly or lightly fermented to produce a nutrient-rich beverage. Fresh sap is high in electrolytes, natural sugars, and trace minerals, making it a suitable drink for hydration, mild energy replenishment, and general vitality. Fermentation with controlled methods yields a mildly effervescent tonic while retaining the nutritional and medicinal qualities of the sap.

Charred Bark Powder for Dental and Hygiene Uses

Charred coconut bark can be powdered and used as a natural dental cleanser or antiseptic. Mix with a small amount of salt or baking soda and use it to gently brush teeth, remove plaque, and strengthen gums. Alternatively, this powder can be incorporated into poultices for minor cuts or skin abrasions to prevent infection and promote healing.

Sustainability and Holistic Integration

These recipes and DIY uses underscore the importance of sustainability and holistic application. Utilizing the trunk and bark ensures minimal waste and maximizes the medicinal potential of the coconut tree. By combining traditional knowledge with practical, modern preparation methods, individuals can access therapeutic benefits while fostering environmentally conscious practices.

In conclusion, coconut trunk and bark can be effectively integrated into culinary, topical, and household preparations, enhancing systemic health, skin care, and hygiene. Their multifunctional use exemplifies the holistic potential of the coconut tree, promoting wellness, sustainability, and practical ingenuity in everyday life.

5: Leaves for Life

5.1 Coconut Leaves: Nutritional and Medicinal Uses

Coconut leaves, commonly regarded as by-products of the tree's fruit-bearing function, possess substantial nutritional and medicinal potential. Ethnobotanical evidence from regions such as South and Southeast Asia, the Pacific Islands, and parts of West Africa highlights their multifaceted applications in traditional medicine, while recent phytochemical analyses provide scientific support for their therapeutic properties.

Traditionally, coconut leaves have been used in the treatment of mild infections, fever, and wounds. Fresh leaf juice is often extracted by pounding young, tender leaves and straining the liquid for oral administration. This juice is employed as a natural diuretic, aiding in the elimination of excess fluid and supporting kidney function. In some Pacific Island cultures, leaf extracts are applied topically to reduce inflammation, treat minor cuts, burns, or insect bites, and soothe skin irritations. Additionally, infusions of dried leaves are sometimes consumed to alleviate fever and gastrointestinal discomfort, illustrating the leaves' dual internal and external medicinal roles.

From a nutritional perspective, coconut leaves contain polyphenols, flavonoids, and essential minerals such as magnesium, calcium, and potassium. These bioactive compounds provide antioxidant, anti-inflammatory, and vasoprotective effects. Flavonoids, in particular, neutralize free radicals and help reduce oxidative stress, while polyphenolic compounds contribute to improved cardiovascular and metabolic health. The mineral content supports electrolyte balance and bone health, indicating that leaf-based preparations can complement dietary intake in regions with limited access to conventional supplements.

Scientific studies have begun to quantify these traditional claims. For example, research in the Journal of Herbal Medicine (2018) demonstrated that aqueous and methanolic extracts of coconut leaves exhibit significant antioxidant activity, inhibit microbial growth, and modulate inflammatory pathways in vitro. These findings corroborate the ethnomedicinal use of leaves for treating infections and inflammation. Additional studies have identified phenolic acids such as ferulic acid, caffeic acid, and gallic acid in leaf extracts, compounds known for their protective effects against oxidative damage and tissue inflammation.

In addition to pharmacological applications, coconut leaves are valued for their nutritional supplementation in traditional diets. In some rural communities, tender leaf extracts are incorporated into soups or broths to fortify meals with trace minerals and antioxidants. This practice reflects an integrated approach to food and medicine, where plants provide both nourishment and preventive health benefits.

Holistically, coconut leaves exemplify the principle of functional plant use, in which a single plant component offers multiple advantages for human well-being. By supporting hydration, antioxidant defense, anti-inflammatory activity, and topical healing, leaves contribute to systemic balance while utilizing a part of the tree that is often discarded or relegated to non-nutritional purposes. Their incorporation into diets, herbal remedies, and topical applications demonstrates the broad therapeutic potential of the coconut beyond its fruit.

In conclusion, coconut leaves represent a valuable, accessible, and underutilized component of the tree. Their nutritional richness, bioactive compounds, and traditional applications establish a foundation for both culinary and medicinal integration. Continued research into standardized preparation methods and dosage optimization will further elucidate their role in holistic health and preventive medicine.

5.2 Preparation and Application of Coconut Leaf Remedies

COCONUT LEAVES OFFER diverse therapeutic benefits that are most effectively realized through proper preparation and application. Traditional and contemporary approaches converge in methods that extract bioactive compounds while preserving their efficacy. This section details techniques for internal consumption, topical use, and functional integration into wellness practices.

Leaf Juice for Internal Use

Fresh, tender coconut leaves are ideal for extracting leaf juice, which functions as a natural diuretic and mild detoxifier. To prepare, clean and wash young leaves thoroughly, then crush or pound them to release the sap. Strain the liquid to obtain a clear juice, which can be consumed in small quantities—typically 50–100 milliliters, one to two times daily. The juice supports kidney function, aids in fluid regulation, and can help alleviate mild fever and urinary discomfort. For enhanced palatability, a small quantity of honey or lime juice may be added without compromising the medicinal properties.

Leaf Decoction for Therapeutic Tonic

For a stronger preparation, dried coconut leaves can be used to make a decoction. Chop 30–50 grams of dried leaves into small pieces and boil in 500 milliliters of water for 15–20 minutes. Strain and consume warm. This decoction delivers higher concentrations of polyphenols and flavonoids, providing antioxidant and anti-inflammatory support.

It is traditionally employed for digestive issues, systemic inflammation, and general revitalization during periods of fatigue or recovery from minor illness.

Topical Applications for Skin and Wound Healing

Coconut leaf extracts can be applied externally to minor cuts, abrasions, insect bites, or inflammatory skin conditions. Fresh leaves can be crushed to obtain a pulp or juice, which is applied directly to the affected area. The combination of polyphenolic compounds and astringent constituents promotes microbial defense, reduces inflammation, and accelerates tissue repair. For additional efficacy, leaf juice may be blended with coconut oil or aloe vera gel to create a soothing topical preparation suitable for sensitive skin.

Leaf Infusions for Bathing and Relaxation

In some traditional practices, coconut leaf infusions are used as part of therapeutic baths. Boil a handful of leaves in water for 10–15 minutes, then add the strained liquid to warm bathwater. This practice provides mild skin cleansing, antioxidant benefits, and a calming effect on the body, supporting holistic relaxation and systemic detoxification.

Integration with Complementary Botanicals

Coconut leaf remedies are often combined with other medicinal plants to enhance their therapeutic effect. For instance, infusion with lemongrass or ginger amplifies anti-inflammatory and antimicrobial action, while addition of lime or honey improves taste and absorption for internal use. Such combinations exemplify synergistic phytotherapy, where multiple plant constituents interact to deliver a broader spectrum of health benefits.

Safety and Dosage Considerations

While generally safe, coconut leaf remedies should be consumed or applied in moderation. Excessive intake of leaf juice may cause mild gastrointestinal discomfort, and topical applications should be tested on a small area to ensure tolerance. Pregnant or lactating individuals should consult healthcare providers before regular use, and all preparations should use clean water and properly sanitized utensils to prevent contamination.

In conclusion, coconut leaf remedies provide versatile and effective means for supporting systemic health and topical healing. Through juicing, decoction, infusion, and topical application, the leaves deliver antioxidant, anti-inflammatory, and antimicrobial benefits, reflecting both traditional wisdom and modern phytochemical validation. Their integration into holistic health practices exemplifies the multifunctionality of the coconut tree as a sustainable and accessible natural resource.

5.3 Recipes and DIY Applications of Coconut Leaves

COCONUT LEAVES OFFER a broad range of culinary and therapeutic applications that extend their utility beyond traditional medicinal uses. By incorporating leaves into recipes and DIY preparations, individuals can leverage their antioxidant, anti-inflammatory, and diuretic properties while promoting sustainability and holistic health. This section presents practical methods for using coconut leaves in daily life.

Coconut Leaf Herbal Tea

A simple and effective preparation involves using fresh or dried leaves to make herbal tea. Wash 30–50 grams of leaves thoroughly and steep them in 500 milliliters of hot water for 10–15 minutes. Strain before consumption. The tea delivers polyphenols, flavonoids, and essential minerals, supporting kidney function, digestive health, and mild systemic detoxification. A small amount of honey or lime can be added to enhance flavor while maintaining therapeutic properties. Regular consumption may contribute to improved energy levels, circulation, and general well-being.

Coconut Leaf Decoction with Ginger and Lemongrass

For enhanced anti-inflammatory and antimicrobial effects, a decoction can be prepared using coconut leaves, fresh ginger, and lemongrass. Boil 50 grams of leaves with a 20-gram piece of ginger and 10 grams of lemongrass in one liter of water for 15–20 minutes. Strain and consume warm. This combination synergistically supports digestive function, immune response, and detoxification pathways, making it suitable for daily wellness or mild illness recovery.

Topical Leaf Paste for Skin Care

Coconut leaves can be made into a topical paste for minor cuts, abrasions, or insect bites. Crush fresh leaves into a pulp and mix with a small quantity of coconut oil to create a smooth paste. Apply directly to affected areas to reduce inflammation and prevent microbial infection. The leaf paste can also be blended with aloe vera gel or turmeric for additional soothing and antiseptic properties, offering a natural, sustainable alternative to commercial skin care products.

Leaf Infusion Bath for Relaxation and Skin Health

Prepare a therapeutic bath infusion by boiling a handful of fresh coconut leaves in water for 10 minutes. Strain the liquid and add it to warm bathwater. Immersing in this infusion provides mild skin cleansing, antioxidant support, and relaxation benefits. This practice aligns with holistic health principles, promoting both physiological and psychological well-being.

Culinary Integration in Soups and Broths

In certain traditional diets, young coconut leaves are incorporated into soups or broths as a nutritional supplement. Tender leaves are cleaned, finely chopped, and added to vegetable-based soups during cooking. This practice enhances the nutrient density of meals, providing essential minerals, antioxidants, and phytochemicals that support systemic health without altering flavor significantly.

Sustainability and Practical Considerations

The use of coconut leaves in recipes and DIY preparations underscores the principle of zero waste. Leaves, which are often discarded, can be repurposed for medicinal, culinary, and hygienic applications, maximizing the tree's utility while promoting environmental responsibility. Proper cleaning, preparation, and storage are essential to maintain efficacy and prevent microbial contamination.

In conclusion, coconut leaves provide versatile avenues for wellness through teas, decoctions, topical pastes, bath infusions, and culinary integration. Their multifunctional properties, when applied thoughtfully, enhance systemic health, support skin care, and encourage sustainable utilization. These practices exemplify the holistic potential of the coconut tree, integrating nutritional, medicinal, and practical benefits into everyday life.

6: The Coconut Flower

6.1 Coconut Fruit: Nutritional Composition and Health Benefits

The coconut fruit (Cocos nucifera L.) is the most widely recognized component of the coconut tree, celebrated for its extensive nutritional profile and versatile health benefits. Comprised of the endosperm (both liquid coconut water and solid kernel), the pericarp, and the husk, the fruit provides macronutrients, micronutrients, and bioactive compounds that support systemic health. Its use spans culinary, medicinal, and functional applications, making it central to both traditional and contemporary health practices.

Nutritional Composition

Coconut fruit exhibits a unique composition of carbohydrates, fats, proteins, vitamins, minerals, and phytonutrients. The solid endosperm, or kernel, contains approximately 33–35% fat, 6–7% protein, and 15–20% carbohydrates, depending on maturity. The fats are predominantly medium-chain triglycerides (MCTs), which are metabolized differently from long-chain fatty acids, offering rapid energy and potential metabolic benefits. Coconut water, the clear liquid endosperm, is low in calories but rich in electrolytes, particularly potassium, sodium, magnesium, and calcium, making it a natural rehydration beverage. Additionally, both the kernel and water contain polyphenols, vitamins C, E, and B-complex, and essential minerals, contributing to antioxidant, anti-inflammatory, and cardioprotective effects.

Health Benefits

The health-promoting properties of coconut fruit are diverse:

1. **Cardiometabolic Support**: The MCTs in coconut kernel are metabolized rapidly, potentially enhancing energy expenditure and supporting weight management. Some studies suggest that MCTs may improve lipid profiles, although the effect is dose-dependent and requires moderation.
2. **Hydration and Electrolyte Balance**: Coconut water provides a natural source of electrolytes and fluid replacement, useful for maintaining hydration during physical exertion or mild dehydration. Its low caloric content and high potassium concentration support cardiovascular function and fluid balance.
3. **Digestive Health**: Dietary fiber in the mature coconut kernel aids gastrointestinal motility, enhances satiety, and supports a healthy microbiome. Additionally, the antimicrobial properties of certain coconut fatty acids, such as lauric acid, may help modulate gut microbial populations.
4. **Antioxidant and Anti-inflammatory Effects**: Both coconut water and kernel contain polyphenolic compounds, which neutralize reactive oxygen species, reducing oxidative stress. Regular consumption can support cellular health, mitigate chronic inflammation, and contribute to overall wellness.
5. **Immune Support**: Lauric acid, capric acid, and other medium-chain fatty acids exhibit antimicrobial and antiviral properties, supporting the body's innate defense mechanisms. These compounds contribute to traditional applications of coconut in preventing and mitigating infections.
6. **Skin and Hair Health**: Coconut oil, derived from the kernel, has been extensively studied for topical applications. It

functions as a moisturizer, barrier enhancer, and antimicrobial agent, promoting skin integrity and scalp health.

Functional Applications

Coconut fruit is incorporated into a variety of culinary and therapeutic formulations, including fresh consumption, dried desiccated coconut, coconut milk, coconut oil, and functional beverages. Its integration into daily diets and medicinal preparations exemplifies the principle of food as medicine, wherein nutrient-dense foods confer both sustenance and health-promoting benefits.

Holistic Perspective

The coconut fruit represents the apex of the tree's multifunctionality, delivering concentrated nutrition and bioactive compounds. Its combination of macronutrients, micronutrients, and phytochemicals provides systemic support, encompassing energy metabolism, hydration, gastrointestinal health, immune function, and skin care. By harnessing both the kernel and water, humans can access a comprehensive range of health benefits while respecting the sustainability of the resource.

In conclusion, the coconut fruit is a nutritionally rich, multifunctional component of Cocos nucifera, offering scientifically supported benefits for metabolic, cardiovascular, gastrointestinal, immune, and dermatological health. Its diverse applications, both dietary and therapeutic, underscore its central role in holistic wellness and its continued relevance in contemporary nutrition and traditional medicine.

6.2 Preparation and Culinary Uses of Coconut Fruit

THE COCONUT FRUIT IS uniquely versatile, with each component—the water, kernel, milk, and oil—capable of contributing to both nutrition and therapeutic applications. Understanding preparation techniques ensures that the bioactive compounds and nutrients are preserved while enhancing palatability and functional utility. This section details methods for incorporating the fruit into culinary practices and health-promoting formulations.

Coconut Water for Hydration and Health

Coconut water is consumed directly from young, tender fruits. Fresh extraction ensures maximum retention of electrolytes, vitamins, and bioactive compounds. For culinary enhancement, it may be chilled and used as a base for natural beverages or smoothies, maintaining its rehydrating and cardiometabolic benefits. Coconut water can also be combined with natural fruit juices to create electrolyte-rich drinks suitable for post-exercise recovery or mild dehydration.

Coconut Kernel Consumption

The white, fleshy kernel of the fruit can be consumed raw, grated, or desiccated. Raw kernels provide dietary fiber, medium-chain triglycerides, and essential micronutrients. Grated or shredded coconut is used in both sweet and savory preparations, such as porridges, curries, and baked goods. Minimal cooking preserves polyphenols and antioxidants, while mature kernels can be dried to produce coconut flour, enhancing the fiber content of various recipes and supporting gastrointestinal health.

Coconut Milk and Cream

Coconut milk and cream are produced by blending grated kernel with water, then straining the mixture to extract a nutrient-dense liquid. Coconut milk is widely used in culinary applications such as soups, stews, sauces, and desserts, providing healthy fats, flavor, and textural richness. The fat content, primarily medium-chain triglycerides, contributes to sustained energy and may support metabolic functions. Coconut cream, being more concentrated, is ideal for rich desserts or therapeutic smoothies where higher fat content is desired.

Coconut Oil Extraction and Use

Coconut oil is derived from the kernel through cold-pressing or heat-mediated extraction. Cold-pressed virgin coconut oil retains most of the antioxidants, polyphenols, and medium-chain fatty acids, offering both dietary and topical benefits. Culinary applications include sautéing, baking, or incorporating into smoothies and salad dressings. For topical use, virgin coconut oil functions as a moisturizer, hair conditioner, and antimicrobial agent, providing a bridge between nutrition and skin/hair therapy.

Traditional and Therapeutic Recipes

Culinary integration of coconut fruit can also serve medicinal purposes. For example, a simple coconut milk and turmeric porridge combines the anti-inflammatory properties of turmeric with the MCTs and antioxidants in coconut, creating a functional food for metabolic and immune support. Similarly, blending fresh coconut water with grated kernel and a small amount of ginger produces a nutrient-rich tonic that hydrates, supports digestion, and delivers antioxidant benefits.

Preservation and Storage

Maintaining nutrient integrity requires careful handling. Coconut water should be consumed soon after extraction or stored in refrigerated conditions for up to 24 hours. Kernels, milk, and cream should be stored in airtight containers at low temperatures to prevent rancidity and microbial growth. Proper storage preserves both the nutritional and therapeutic qualities of the fruit.

Holistic Application

The coconut fruit exemplifies the concept of food as medicine. Its versatile preparation methods allow for dietary integration, functional beverages, and therapeutic formulations that promote systemic health. Through careful extraction, minimal processing, and thoughtful culinary design, the coconut fruit delivers a wide array of benefits spanning metabolic, cardiovascular, gastrointestinal, immune, and dermatological health.

In summary, the preparation and culinary use of coconut fruit maximize its nutritional density and therapeutic potential. By leveraging water, kernel, milk, and oil, individuals can create meals, beverages, and functional remedies that support holistic well-being, reflecting both traditional wisdom and modern nutritional science.

6.3 Recipes and DIY Applications of Coconut Fruit

Coconut fruit, encompassing the water, kernel, milk, and oil, offers extensive opportunities for both culinary and therapeutic applications. Proper utilization allows for the creation of nutrient-rich recipes and DIY preparations that enhance systemic health, support wellness routines, and exemplify the functional integration of food and medicine. This section provides practical methods for maximizing the benefits of the coconut fruit.

Coconut Water-Based Recipes

Coconut water can be consumed directly or combined with fruits and natural sweeteners to produce hydrating and antioxidant-rich beverages. A simple recipe involves blending 250 milliliters of coconut water with half a banana, a few slices of pineapple, and a teaspoon of honey to create a nutrient-dense smoothie. This preparation supports hydration, electrolyte balance, and digestive health while providing antioxidants and natural energy.

Coconut Kernel Preparations

he white kernel can be incorporated into meals as raw shreds, grated additions, or dried flour. A traditional therapeutic preparation is a coconut porridge, made by boiling 100 grams of grated kernel with water and a small amount of turmeric or ginger. This porridge provides dietary fiber, medium-chain triglycerides, and anti-inflammatory compounds, serving as both a nourishing meal and a functional tonic. Grated coconut can also be added to salads, soups, or baked goods to enhance nutritional density.

Coconut Milk and Cream Recipes

Coconut milk and cream can be used to prepare nutrient-dense dishes with both culinary and therapeutic benefits. For example, a coconut milk and vegetable stew combines 200 milliliters of coconut milk with assorted vegetables and mild spices, providing antioxidants, minerals, and healthy fats that support digestion and systemic energy. Similarly, coconut cream blended with fruits and a small amount of honey or date syrup can serve as a functional dessert that delivers anti-inflammatory and metabolic benefits.

DIY Coconut Oil Applications

Coconut oil, extracted from the kernel, serves both dietary and topical purposes. For cooking, virgin coconut oil can be used in sautéing vegetables or in baked goods, preserving medium-chain triglycerides and antioxidants. Topically, coconut oil can be combined with essential oils, aloe vera, or powdered herbs to create moisturizers, hair conditioners, or antimicrobial ointments. This dual application underscores the multifunctionality of the coconut fruit in promoting wellness through internal and external use.

Coconut Fruit Functional Tonics

Combining different parts of the coconut fruit into a single preparation amplifies health benefits. For instance, a functional tonic can be created by blending 100 milliliters of coconut water with 50 grams of grated kernel and a teaspoon of grated ginger. Consumed in the morning, this tonic provides hydration, antioxidants, electrolytes, and anti-inflammatory compounds, supporting systemic resilience and overall vitality.

Sustainability and Resource Efficiency

The use of coconut fruit in recipes and DIY preparations emphasizes sustainability and holistic resource utilization. Each component—the water, kernel, milk, and oil—can be applied to promote nutrition, health, and wellness, minimizing waste while maximizing therapeutic and culinary potential.

In conclusion, coconut fruit offers an extensive array of applications that bridge nutrition and medicine. Through beverages, porridges, stews, desserts, and topical formulations, individuals can harness the full spectrum of bioactive compounds and nutrients, reinforcing the coconut's role as a multifunctional resource for holistic health and sustainable living.

7: Integrative Health Applications of the Coconut Plant

7.1 Integrating Coconut Plant Components into a Holistic Wellness Routine

The comprehensive use of the coconut plant—from roots, trunk, and bark, to leaves and fruit—illustrates the potential for a fully integrated approach to health and wellness. Each part of the plant contributes unique bioactive compounds and nutritional benefits, allowing for the development of routines that support systemic balance, disease prevention, and holistic vitality. Integrating these components thoughtfully into daily life maximizes their therapeutic potential while promoting sustainable utilization.

Designing a Daily Wellness Routine

A holistic coconut-based wellness routine can be structured around the unique properties of each plant component. For example, morning hydration may begin with fresh coconut water, providing electrolytes and supporting kidney function. Mid-morning intake could include a small serving of coconut leaf tea or decoction, supplying antioxidants and promoting digestive health. Meals may incorporate grated coconut kernel, coconut milk, or coconut flour, offering medium-chain triglycerides, dietary fiber, and essential minerals to sustain energy and metabolic balance. Throughout the day, topical applications of coconut oil or bark/leaf pastes can support skin integrity, reduce microbial exposure, and provide anti-inflammatory effects.

Synergistic Combinations for Enhanced Benefits

Integrating multiple components can enhance the overall health impact. For instance, a morning smoothie combining coconut water, grated kernel, and a small quantity of young leaf extract delivers hydration, antioxidants, fiber, and essential nutrients in a single preparation. Similarly, a therapeutic soup incorporating coconut milk, grated kernel, and bark or leaf decoctions can provide both nutritive and medicinal effects, supporting gastrointestinal health, metabolic regulation, and immune function.

Seasonal and Contextual Adaptations

The holistic integration of coconut components may be tailored according to seasonal and environmental conditions. During periods of heat or high physical activity, emphasis on coconut water and leaf tea can enhance hydration and electrolyte replenishment. In colder or more sedentary periods, incorporating coconut milk-based soups or porridges provides sustained energy and metabolic support. This flexibility ensures that the wellness routine is adaptive, practical, and aligned with individual physiological needs.

Preventive and Restorative Health Applications

Coconut plant-based routines can serve both preventive and restorative purposes. Regular consumption of coconut water, kernel, and leaf teas supports systemic detoxification, antioxidant defense, and metabolic balance, contributing to disease prevention. Topical applications of coconut oil, bark, and leaf pastes facilitate tissue repair, antimicrobial defense, and skin health, supporting recovery from minor injuries or inflammatory conditions. Such a routine underscores the principle of holistic wellness, integrating both internal and external health-promoting strategies.

Practical Implementation Guidelines

To optimize the benefits of coconut-based wellness routines, certain practical considerations should be observed:

1. Use fresh, clean, and minimally processed plant components to preserve bioactive compounds.
2. Incorporate a variety of components throughout the day to ensure broad-spectrum nutritional and therapeutic coverage.
3. Monitor individual tolerance to specific preparations, adjusting dosage and frequency as needed.
4. Maintain hygienic preparation methods for all topical and ingestible applications to prevent contamination.
5. Combine coconut-based interventions with other lifestyle measures such as balanced nutrition, adequate sleep, and regular physical activity for comprehensive wellness.

Holistic Perspective

The systematic incorporation of coconut plant components exemplifies a model of integrative wellness, where food, medicine, and daily care converge. By leveraging the unique attributes of roots, trunk, bark, leaves, and fruit, individuals can create routines that not only nourish but also protect, restore, and sustain health. This approach emphasizes the synergy between plant-based bioactive compounds and daily lifestyle practices, promoting resilience, vitality, and holistic well-being.

In summary, a holistic wellness routine centered on the coconut plant provides a practical framework for integrating nutrition, herbal medicine, and topical care into daily life. Such routines harness the full spectrum of the plant's bioactive potential, aligning traditional knowledge with modern understanding to support systemic health, preventative care, and sustainable resource use.

7.2 Designing Daily Coconut-Based Health

and Nutrition Plans

THE CREATION OF STRUCTURED daily health and nutrition plans using coconut plant components allows individuals to systematically harness the plant's therapeutic, nutritional, and functional properties. Such plans integrate evidence-based consumption patterns, timing, and preparation methods to optimize health outcomes while fostering sustainability and holistic well-being.

Morning Routine

The day may begin with hydration and gentle detoxification using coconut water, which replenishes electrolytes, supports kidney function, and provides low-calorie hydration. Supplementing this with a small quantity of young leaf extract or tea enhances antioxidant intake and prepares the digestive system for the day. For individuals seeking an energy boost, blending coconut water with grated kernel, a touch of natural sweetener, and a small piece of ginger can serve as a functional morning tonic.

Midday Nutrition

Meals incorporating coconut kernel, coconut milk, or coconut flour provide sustained energy and medium-chain triglycerides, supporting metabolism and satiety. For example, a coconut milk-based vegetable stew or a porridge enriched with grated kernel and spices such as turmeric offers antioxidants, minerals, and anti-inflammatory compounds. Coconut flour can be used in baking or meal preparations to increase fiber content and maintain digestive regularity. Integrating leaf decoctions as a beverage with lunch enhances nutrient intake and promotes systemic antioxidant defense.

Afternoon Wellness and Snacks

To maintain energy and hydration during the afternoon, coconut water-based smoothies or light snacks incorporating grated coconut can provide sustained metabolic support and micronutrients. This may include blending coconut water with fresh fruits or preparing small coconut leaf infusions. Such practices help regulate blood sugar, maintain hydration, and support cognitive function.

Evening and Topical Applications

Evening routines can focus on restorative and preventive care. Topical application of coconut oil or bark and leaf pastes to the skin or scalp supports repair, hydration, and antimicrobial protection. Coconut milk or kernel-based soups can serve as a light, nutrient-dense dinner, promoting digestion and providing sustained energy overnight. Herbal infusions from leaves or bark may be consumed as warm beverages to aid relaxation, reduce systemic inflammation, and promote restorative sleep.

Customization and Individualization

Coconut-based nutrition and health plans can be tailored according to age, physiological needs, activity levels, and health status. For example, athletes may require additional coconut water and kernel intake for energy and electrolyte replenishment, while individuals with inflammatory conditions may benefit from higher frequency of leaf or bark decoctions. Adjusting portion sizes, combinations, and preparation methods ensures that the routine remains safe, effective, and aligned with individual health objectives.

Integration with Broader Lifestyle Practices

Optimal outcomes are achieved when coconut-based plans are integrated with complementary lifestyle practices. Balanced diet choices, regular physical activity, stress management techniques, and adequate sleep amplify the benefits of coconut-derived nutrients and bioactive compounds. Such integration reflects a holistic approach to wellness, where food, herbal medicine, and daily habits converge to sustain systemic health.

Sustainability Considerations

By incorporating all components of the coconut plant into daily routines, these plans also promote sustainable resource utilization. Roots, trunk, bark, leaves, and fruit can each contribute to nutrition, hydration, topical care, and functional remedies, minimizing waste and emphasizing eco-conscious wellness practices.

In conclusion, daily health and nutrition plans utilizing coconut plant components provide a structured, adaptable, and holistic framework for promoting systemic wellness. Through strategic timing, thoughtful preparation, and synergistic integration of roots, trunk, bark, leaves, and fruit, individuals can harness the full spectrum of the coconut's nutritional and therapeutic potential, supporting long-term vitality, preventive care, and sustainable living.

7.3 Sample Weekly Coconut-Based Wellness Plan with Recipes

IMPLEMENTING A STRUCTURED, week-long wellness plan utilizing coconut plant components allows individuals to systematically integrate nutrition, herbal remedies, and topical care into their daily routine. This plan emphasizes the multifunctional properties of coconut roots, trunk, bark, leaves, and fruit, combining traditional knowledge with modern nutritional science. Below is a sample framework adaptable to different lifestyles and health objectives.

Day 1: Hydration and Antioxidant Support

- **Morning**: Consume 250 milliliters of fresh coconut water with a teaspoon of grated young leaf juice. This provides electrolytes, hydration, and antioxidants to start the day.
- **Midday:** Prepare a coconut milk vegetable stew containing 100 milliliters of coconut milk, assorted vegetables, and a pinch of turmeric. Consume alongside a small serving of grated coconut kernel.
- **Afternoon**: Drink a light coconut leaf infusion or tea to support systemic detoxification.
- **Evening:** Topically apply a paste made from coconut leaf juice and virgin coconut oil to minor skin irritations or dry areas.

Day 2: Digestive Health and Metabolic Support

- **Morning**: Blend coconut water with grated coconut kernel, a slice of ginger, and a teaspoon of honey to make a functional smoothie that supports digestion and provides energy.
- **Midday:** Eat a coconut flour-based porridge or baked dish enriched with vegetables or legumes, supplying fiber, minerals, and medium-chain triglycerides.
- **Afternoon:** Drink a warm bark decoction prepared from 30 grams of dried trunk bark to promote gastrointestinal health.\
- **Evening:** Coconut oil massage for skin hydration and relaxation, or apply leaf and bark paste to support topical healing.

Day 3: Anti-Inflammatory Focus

- **Morning**: Coconut leaf tea infused with lemongrass or ginger, enhancing anti-inflammatory effects.
- **Midday**: Coconut milk-based curry or soup incorporating spices like turmeric and black pepper, with grated kernel for added fiber and fats.

- **Afternoon:** Snack on fresh grated coconut or a coconut water-based smoothie.
- **Evening**: Topical application of a bark and leaf paste on areas of minor inflammation or insect bites.

Day 4: Energy and Electrolyte Replenishment

- **Morning**: Drink 250 milliliters of fresh coconut water and consume a small portion of tender leaf juice.
- **Midday**: Coconut milk vegetable stew with added protein (legumes or lean meat) for sustained energy.
- **Afternoon**: Coconut water-based fruit smoothie or a coconut leaf tea.
- **Evening**: Coconut oil topical application, and, if desired, a mild leaf infusion before bedtime for relaxation.

Day 5: Immune and Antioxidant Support

Morning: Blend coconut water with grated kernel, honey, and a small amount of turmeric for an immune-boosting tonic.

Midday: Consume a coconut flour-based dish or porridge enriched with spices and vegetables.

Afternoon: Drink a bark or leaf decoction to enhance antioxidant intake.

Evening: Apply coconut oil and leaf paste topically as part of a restorative skin routine.

Day 6: Hydration and Digestive Wellness

Morning: Coconut water with young leaf juice for hydration and mild detoxification.

Midday: Coconut milk vegetable stew with grated kernel. Optionally add legumes for fiber.

Afternoon: Coconut leaf tea or a light smoothie with coconut water and fruit.

Evening: Topical coconut oil application for skin hydration and antimicrobial protection.

Day 7: Restorative and Holistic Care

Morning: Coconut water-based smoothie with grated kernel and a small piece of ginger.

Midday: Coconut milk-based soup with vegetables and optional bark decoction incorporated.

Afternoon: Coconut leaf tea for systemic relaxation and antioxidant support.

Evening: Full topical application of coconut oil, leaf, and bark paste as a holistic skin and tissue restorative measure.

Implementation Notes

- Quantities can be adjusted based on age, activity level, and health status.
- Fresh, minimally processed coconut components should be prioritized for maximal nutrient and bioactive retention.
- Hygiene and preparation standards are essential to prevent contamination and preserve efficacy.
- Recipes can be adapted seasonally or according to local ingredient availability.

Holistic Perspective

This sample weekly plan illustrates the integration of coconut plant components into a comprehensive wellness routine. By combining hydration, nutrition, topical care, and functional herbal preparations, individuals can support digestive, metabolic, immune, and dermatological health. Moreover, the plan demonstrates sustainable use of all parts of the coconut plant, fostering resource efficiency and holistic well-being.

In conclusion, a structured weekly wellness routine based on coconut plant components serves as a practical, adaptable, and scientifically informed approach to holistic health, merging traditional practices with contemporary nutritional and medicinal insights.

8: Sustainability, Standardization, and Safe Use of Coconut-Based Products

8.1 Safety, Dosage, and Contraindications of Coconut Plant Applications

While the coconut plant (Cocos nucifera L.) offers extensive nutritional, medicinal, and functional benefits, the proper use of its components requires attention to safety, dosage, and potential contraindications. Understanding these factors ensures that consumers can maximize health outcomes while minimizing adverse effects, particularly when integrating roots, trunk, bark, leaves, and fruit into daily routines.

General Safety Considerations

Coconut plant components are generally considered safe for consumption and topical use when prepared appropriately. Hygiene and proper cleaning of plant parts are essential to prevent microbial contamination, especially for fresh leaves, bark, and coconut water. Use of clean utensils and containers, and avoiding prolonged storage at room temperature, reduces the risk of foodborne illness. Topical applications should be applied to small skin areas initially to assess sensitivity, particularly for individuals with a history of skin allergies.

Recommended Dosage Guidelines

Coconut Water: 200–300 milliliters per serving is typically sufficient for hydration and electrolyte replenishment. Excessive consumption may lead to mild gastrointestinal discomfort or electrolyte imbalance in sensitive individuals.

Coconut Kernel: Daily intake of 30–50 grams, grated or shredded, is generally safe for most adults, providing dietary fiber and medium-chain triglycerides without excessive caloric load.

Coconut Milk and Cream: Moderate consumption (100–200 milliliters per meal) ensures nutrient intake without overloading dietary fats.

Coconut Oil: For dietary purposes, 1–2 tablespoons per day is usually adequate; topical application may be done once or twice daily as needed.

Leaves, Bark, and Roots: Herbal decoctions or infusions are generally consumed in moderate quantities—50–100 milliliters per dose, up to 2–3 times daily. Topical pastes should be applied thinly, and frequency adjusted according to skin tolerance.

Potential Contraindications

- Individuals with known allergies to coconut or tree nuts should avoid ingestion or topical application.
- Excessive intake of coconut water may be contraindicated in individuals with kidney dysfunction or hyperkalemia due to high potassium content.
- Coconut oil should be used with caution in patients with specific lipid disorders or cardiovascular risk factors if consumed in large quantities.
- Pregnant or lactating individuals should consult healthcare professionals before regular consumption of concentrated herbal decoctions derived from leaves, bark, or roots.
- Topical preparations may cause irritation or allergic reactions in sensitive skin; patch testing is recommended before full application.

Drug and Food Interactions

Certain coconut plant applications may interact with medications or dietary supplements:

1. Coconut water, due to high potassium levels, may interact with potassium-sparing diuretics, ACE inhibitors, or other medications affecting electrolyte balance.
2. Coconut oil, when consumed in large quantities, may influence lipid-lowering medications or weight management plans.
3. Herbal extracts from leaves, bark, or roots may interact with anticoagulants, anti-inflammatory drugs, or other herbal supplements, depending on bioactive compound profiles. Consultation with a healthcare professional is advisable for individuals on chronic medication.

Special Populations

Children, elderly individuals, and those with chronic health conditions should use coconut-based preparations with caution, adjusting portion sizes and frequency according to physiological needs and tolerances. Monitoring for adverse effects, such as gastrointestinal upset, skin reactions, or unusual fatigue, is recommended.

Holistic Safety Perspective

Coconut plant applications exemplify the principle of functional food and herbal medicine integration. While generally safe, responsible usage—including attention to hygiene, dosage, individual health status, and potential interactions—ensures that benefits are maximized while minimizing risk. Education on proper preparation, consumption, and topical application reinforces both therapeutic efficacy and safety.

In conclusion, the safe and effective use of coconut plant components requires attention to recommended dosages, awareness of contraindications, and consideration of individual health circumstances. When applied responsibly, coconut-based nutrition and wellness practices can provide substantial health benefits across multiple physiological systems.

8.2 Best Practices for Preparing and Storing Coconut Plant Materials

THE EFFICACY OF COCONUT plant applications is closely linked to proper preparation and storage. Each component—roots, trunk, bark, leaves, and fruit—contains sensitive bioactive compounds that can degrade under poor handling conditions. Implementing best practices ensures the preservation of nutritional and medicinal properties, enhances safety, and supports long-term sustainability.

General Preparation Guidelines

- **Cleaning:** All plant materials should be thoroughly rinsed under clean, running water to remove dirt, debris, and potential microbial contaminants. This step is essential for leaves, bark, roots, and the coconut fruit.
- **Trimming and Peeling**: Remove any damaged or decayed portions of roots, bark, or leaves. For fruit, husk removal and separation of water and kernel should be done carefully to prevent contamination.
- **Cutting and Shredding**: Standardize cutting sizes for leaves, bark, or kernels to facilitate consistent extraction of bioactive compounds during decoction, infusion, or culinary preparation. Finely grated kernels and uniformly chopped leaves enhance flavor, nutrient availability, and extract efficiency.

Extraction Techniques

- **Decoction:** Boil dried or fresh plant components in water to extract soluble bioactive compounds. Maintain gentle heat to avoid degradation of heat-sensitive constituents. Strain solids before consumption.
- **Infusion**: Steep leaves or bark in hot water for 10–15 minutes to extract antioxidants and polyphenols without prolonged heating. This method preserves delicate phytochemicals.
- **Juicing:** Crush young leaves or tender roots and strain to obtain juice, which delivers concentrated nutrients. Immediate consumption or proper refrigeration is recommended to prevent microbial growth.
- **Oil Extraction**: Cold-press or minimally heat virgin coconut oil to retain medium-chain triglycerides, antioxidants, and phenolic compounds. Avoid excessive heat or chemical solvents to preserve quality.

Storage Best Practices

- **Refrigeration**: Fresh coconut water, leaf juice, and grated kernel should be stored in airtight containers at 4–6°C and consumed within 24–48 hours.
- **Drying**: Leaves, bark, and roots intended for decoction or infusion can be air-dried or oven-dried at low temperatures (40–50°C) to reduce moisture content and prevent mold growth. Properly dried materials can be stored for several months.
- **Freezing:** Coconut water, grated kernel, and leaf extracts can be frozen for longer-term storage. Thaw gently to preserve nutrient integrity.
- **Containers:** Use clean, food-grade containers made of glass or stainless steel. Avoid plastic containers that may leach

chemicals or absorb odors.

- **Labeling:** Clearly label all stored materials with the date of preparation, type of component, and intended use. This practice prevents spoilage, ensures proper rotation, and maintains quality.

Hygiene and Handling

- Wash hands thoroughly before handling plant materials.

- Use sanitized knives, cutting boards, and utensils to reduce contamination risk.

- Avoid prolonged exposure to sunlight or humid environments, which can degrade phytochemicals and promote microbial growth.
- For topical applications, ensure that pastes, oils, or decoctions are prepared in a clean environment to maintain safety and efficacy.

Sustainability Considerations

Efficient preparation and storage minimize waste by extending the shelf-life of plant components and allowing their full utilization in culinary, medicinal, and wellness applications. By optimizing handling and storage, users can integrate coconut plant components into daily routines without compromising quality or therapeutic benefits.

Holistic Perspective

Adhering to best practices in preparation and storage ensures that the nutritional, medicinal, and functional potential of the coconut plant is fully realized. Proper handling preserves bioactive compounds, safeguards health, and supports sustainable use of all plant components, from roots and bark to leaves and fruit.

In conclusion, meticulous preparation and storage of coconut plant materials are essential for maximizing safety, efficacy, and longevity. Implementing standardized methods allows for consistent integration of coconut-based nutrition, therapeutics, and topical applications into daily life, aligning traditional knowledge with modern health practices.

9: Research Gaps, Innovations, and Future Directions in Coconut Science

9.1 Research Gaps and Future Directions in Coconut Plant Applications

Despite extensive traditional knowledge and emerging scientific evidence supporting the health and functional benefits of Cocos nucifera L., significant research gaps remain. Addressing these gaps is essential to optimize the therapeutic potential, inform public health recommendations, and advance sustainable utilization practices.

Limited Clinical Evidence

While in vitro and animal studies suggest that coconut components possess antimicrobial, anti-inflammatory, antioxidant, and metabolic benefits, there is a scarcity of rigorous clinical trials validating these effects in humans. Systematic investigations evaluating dosage, bioavailability, and long-term outcomes are necessary to substantiate therapeutic claims, particularly for leaf decoctions, bark extracts, and root preparations.

Bioactive Compound Characterization

Although medium-chain triglycerides (MCTs), polyphenols, flavonoids, and lauric acid are identified as key bioactive constituents, comprehensive profiling of all coconut plant components—including leaves, roots, and bark—is limited. Advanced analytical techniques such as high-performance liquid chromatography (HPLC) and mass spectrometry could enhance understanding of bioactive compound composition, synergistic interactions, and stability under different preparation methods.

Standardization of Preparations

Traditional and contemporary uses of coconut plant materials vary widely in preparation methods, concentrations, and dosages. This variability hampers reproducibility, safety assessment, and efficacy evaluation. Developing standardized protocols for decoctions, infusions, pastes, and culinary applications is critical to ensure consistent therapeutic outcomes and facilitate integration into evidence-based practices.

Safety and Toxicological Studies

Comprehensive toxicological studies examining the long-term consumption or topical application of all coconut plant components are limited. While generally considered safe, systematic evaluation of potential interactions with medications, high-dose consumption effects, and safety in special populations (children, elderly, pregnant or lactating individuals) remains an important research priority.

Functional Food and Nutraceutical Development

There is untapped potential for the development of functional foods, nutraceuticals, and integrated wellness products derived from coconut plant components. Research is needed to optimize formulation, assess stability, bioavailability, and efficacy, and explore consumer acceptability. This would bridge traditional knowledge with modern food science and commercial application.

Environmental and Sustainability Research

Sustainable harvesting, processing, and utilization of all coconut plant components—especially leaves, bark, and roots—requires further investigation. Studies on agroforestry practices, waste minimization, and value-added product development can inform environmentally responsible and economically viable strategies.

Public Health and Nutrition Studies

Despite widespread use in tropical regions, limited epidemiological data exists on the impact of regular coconut consumption and topical applications on population health outcomes. Longitudinal studies assessing metabolic, cardiovascular, gastrointestinal, and dermatological impacts would provide valuable evidence to guide public health recommendations.

Future Directions

Future research should focus on:

- Conducting controlled clinical trials to validate traditional claims and quantify health benefits.
- Characterizing bioactive compounds in all plant components and understanding their synergistic effects.
- Developing standardized preparation and dosing protocols for therapeutic, culinary, and topical applications.
- Evaluating safety, tolerability, and potential interactions in diverse populations.
- Innovating functional foods, nutraceuticals, and holistic wellness products leveraging all plant parts.
- Promoting sustainable utilization practices to minimize waste and maximize resource efficiency.
- Integrating traditional knowledge with modern scientific approaches to enhance evidence-based application and community health impact.

Holistic Perspective

Advancing research on coconut plant applications aligns traditional ethnobotanical knowledge with contemporary science, fostering the development of sustainable, safe, and efficacious interventions. Bridging these gaps will facilitate the integration of coconut-based strategies into nutrition, medicine, and holistic wellness, while supporting ecological and socio-economic sustainability.

In conclusion, addressing research gaps in coconut plant applications presents opportunities to validate traditional practices, optimize health outcomes, and support the development of innovative, sustainable, and evidence-based wellness strategies.

9.2 Potential Innovations and Commercial Applications

THE COCONUT PLANT (Cocos nucifera L.) offers extensive opportunities for innovation across nutrition, wellness, therapeutics, and commercial industries. By leveraging its multifunctional components—roots, trunk, bark, leaves, and fruit—entrepreneurs, researchers, and communities can create products and interventions that deliver health benefits, support sustainable livelihoods, and integrate traditional knowledge with modern technologies.

Functional Foods and Nutraceuticals

Coconut fruit and derived products, including water, kernel, milk, cream, and oil, can be incorporated into functional foods and nutraceuticals. Innovations include fortified beverages, energy bars, coconut flour-based baked goods, and protein supplements enriched with coconut MCTs and antioxidants. Research-driven formulations may target cardiovascular health, metabolic regulation, digestive support, and immune enhancement, translating traditional benefits into evidence-based commercial products.

Herbal Extracts and Therapeutic Preparations

Leaves, bark, and roots contain bioactive compounds with antimicrobial, antioxidant, and anti-inflammatory properties. Standardized herbal extracts, decoctions, and topical formulations can be developed for commercial distribution as wellness teas, ointments, balms, or skincare products. Such products capitalize on the plant's therapeutic properties while adhering to safety, dosage, and quality standards.

Cosmetic and Personal Care Products

Virgin coconut oil, leaf extracts, and bark-based pastes can be integrated into cosmetic and personal care products. Potential applications include moisturizers, hair conditioners, anti-inflammatory creams, and natural antimicrobial agents. These products cater to consumers seeking natural, plant-based alternatives, and provide opportunities for branding around sustainability and traditional botanical knowledge.

Agro-Processing and Value-Added Products

Beyond direct consumption, coconut plant components can be transformed into value-added products that enhance economic sustainability. Examples include dried leaf powders for teas, bark-based herbal supplements, coconut shell-based activated carbon, and fiber from husks for textiles or packaging. By diversifying product lines, communities can generate income while utilizing all parts of the plant efficiently.

Innovative Culinary Applications

Culinary innovation includes integrating coconut derivatives into modern gastronomy, plant-based diets, and health-focused meal plans. This may involve novel recipes, fortified foods, smoothies, and dietary supplements that preserve the bioactive properties of coconut while appealing to contemporary consumer preferences.

Integration with Digital Health and Wellness

Digital platforms can support the dissemination of coconut-based wellness programs, recipes, and therapeutic interventions. Mobile applications, online courses, and virtual coaching can educate consumers on daily routines, preparation techniques, and safety protocols, enhancing adoption and adherence while bridging knowledge gaps.

Sustainability and Circular Economy Approaches

Commercial applications must prioritize sustainability to reduce waste and environmental impact. Utilizing all plant components—from roots to leaves to fruit—encourages a circular economy model, where by-products are repurposed into functional or commercial items. This approach not only maximizes economic value but also promotes environmental stewardship.

Research-Driven Product Development

Scientific research underpins product innovation by validating bioactive properties, optimizing preparation methods, and assessing safety and efficacy. Collaborations between academia, industry, and traditional practitioners can accelerate the development of commercially viable products that are both evidence-based and culturally informed.

Holistic Perspective

The multifunctional nature of the coconut plant allows for the integration of nutrition, therapeutics, cosmetics, and sustainability into coherent commercial strategies. Innovations grounded in science, cultural knowledge, and ecological responsibility can support health, community livelihoods, and market expansion simultaneously.

In conclusion, potential innovations and commercial applications of the coconut plant span functional foods, nutraceuticals, herbal therapeutics, cosmetics, value-added products, and digital health integration. Harnessing these opportunities requires a careful balance of traditional knowledge, scientific validation, safety considerations, and sustainable practices, positioning the coconut as a versatile resource for both wellness and economic development.

10: Concluding Remarks on Coconut Plant Utilization and Holistic Health

The coconut plant (Cocos nucifera L.) represents a uniquely versatile botanical resource with significant implications for nutrition, medicine, wellness, and sustainable development. Its diverse components—including roots, trunk, bark, leaves, and fruit—offer bioactive compounds, essential nutrients, and functional properties that can be integrated into daily life to support systemic health and holistic well-being.

Integration of Nutritional and Therapeutic Benefits

Throughout this text, evidence demonstrates that coconut components contribute to cardiovascular, metabolic, gastrointestinal, immune, and dermatological health. Coconut water provides hydration and electrolytes; kernels supply fiber and medium-chain triglycerides; milk and cream deliver fats and bioactive compounds; leaves, bark, and roots contribute antioxidants, anti-inflammatory agents, and other phytonutrients. Proper preparation, dosage, and utilization allow these benefits to be harnessed effectively, bridging traditional knowledge with modern nutritional and medicinal practices.

Holistic Wellness Applications

A holistic approach emphasizes the concurrent use of multiple plant components in daily routines, functional meals, beverages, and topical formulations. Structured wellness plans and weekly schedules enable individuals to integrate hydration, nutrition, herbal remedies, and skin care seamlessly. This integrative model demonstrates how food, medicine, and lifestyle converge to promote preventive and restorative health.

Safety, Standardization, and Sustainability

The safe and effective use of coconut components requires attention to hygiene, storage, preparation methods, and dosage. Standardized protocols for extraction, cooking, decoctions, infusions, and topical applications enhance efficacy while minimizing risks. Sustainable utilization of all plant parts—from roots and bark to leaves and fruit—reduces waste and supports environmental stewardship, reflecting the broader principles of circular economy and eco-conscious wellness practices.

Research and Innovation Potential

Despite extensive traditional and contemporary knowledge, gaps remain in clinical validation, bioactive compound characterization, and safety evaluation. Future research should focus on human trials, functional food development, standardization, and sustainable commercial applications. Innovations in nutraceuticals, cosmetics, culinary applications, and digital wellness platforms present opportunities to expand the reach of coconut-based health strategies.

Holistic Perspective

The coconut plant exemplifies the integration of nutrition, medicine, and wellness in a sustainable and culturally relevant framework. Its multifaceted applications demonstrate that a single botanical resource can address diverse physiological, therapeutic, and lifestyle needs, reinforcing the value of plant-based interventions in contemporary health paradigms.

Final Reflections

Harnessing the full potential of the coconut plant requires a synergistic approach that combines scientific validation, traditional knowledge, structured wellness planning, and sustainable commercial practices. By systematically integrating its nutritional, medicinal, and functional properties into daily life, individuals and communities can achieve enhanced health, preventive care, and holistic well-being, while contributing to economic and ecological sustainability. The coconut thus serves as a model for plant-based holistic health, illustrating the profound impact of natural resources when utilized responsibly and knowledgeably.

Appendices

Appendix A – Additional Recipes, DIY Guides, and Preparation Tables for Coconut Plant Applications

This appendix provides supplemental resources to enhance the practical application of the coconut plant (Cocos nucifera L.) in nutrition, wellness, and topical care. It includes detailed recipes, DIY guides, and preparation tables for various plant components, supporting integration into daily routines.

A.1 Additional Recipes

1. Coconut and Ginger Immune Booster Smoothie

- **Ingredients:** 200 ml coconut water, 50 g grated coconut kernel, 1 tsp grated ginger, 1 tsp honey.
- **Preparation:** Blend all ingredients until smooth. Consume in the morning to support immunity, hydration, and digestion.

1. Coconut Leaf Detox Tea

- **Ingredients:** 5–6 fresh young leaves, 250 ml boiling water.
- **Preparation**: Rinse leaves thoroughly, steep in boiling water for 10 minutes, strain, and consume warm. Supports antioxidant intake and mild detoxification.

1. Coconut Milk Vegetable Soup

- **Ingredients:** 200 ml coconut milk, assorted vegetables

(carrots, spinach, beans), pinch of turmeric, salt to taste.

- **Preparation**: Sauté vegetables lightly, add coconut milk and spices, simmer for 10–15 minutes. Provides fiber, healthy fats, and anti-inflammatory compounds.

1. Coconut Oil Hair Conditioner

- **Ingredients**: 2 tbsp virgin coconut oil, 5 drops essential oil (optional).
- **Preparation:** Warm coconut oil slightly, massage into scalp and hair, leave for 30–60 minutes, then rinse. Supports hair hydration and scalp health.

1. Bark and Leaf Antimicrobial Paste

- **Ingredients**: 2 tbsp powdered bark, 2 tbsp leaf juice, 1 tsp coconut oil.
- **Preparation**: Mix to form a smooth paste. Apply to minor cuts or insect bites to reduce microbial risk and inflammation.

A.2 DIY Guides

1. Coconut Milk Extraction

- Grate fresh kernel.
- Add 200 ml warm water per 100 g kernel.
- Blend and strain through a fine mesh or cheesecloth.
- Fresh milk can be stored in a refrigerated container for 24 hours.

1. Leaf Decoction Preparation

- Rinse and chop fresh leaves.

- Boil 30 g leaves in 500 ml water for 10–15 minutes.
- Strain before consumption. Can be taken up to 2–3 times daily.

1. Coconut Oil Cold-Press Method (Small Scale)

- Grate mature kernel.
- Dry or lightly warm to reduce moisture.
- Press using a manual or mechanical press to extract oil.
- Store in a clean, airtight glass container in a cool place.

A.3 Preparation Tables for Coconut Plant Components

Component	Preparation Method	Recommended Dosage/Use	Storage Guidance
Coconut water	Fresh extraction	200–300 ml per serving	Refrigerate 24–48 hours
Kernel	Grated, shredded, dried	30–50 g per day	Airtight container, cool dry place
Coconut milk/cream	Blending and straining	100–200 ml per meal	Refrigerate 24–48 hours
Coconut oil	Cold-press or minimal heat extraction	1–2 tbsp/day dietary; 1–2x daily topical	Airtight, cool, dark container
Leaves	Decoction, infusion, juice	50–100 ml per dose; 2–3x daily	Refrigerate fresh juice;
Bark	Powder, decoction	50–100 ml decoction; up to 2–3x daily	Refrigerate fris: dried roots 6–12 months

A.4 PRACTICAL TIPS

- Always prioritize fresh, clean, and minimally processed plant materials.
- Standardize preparation quantities to ensure consistent nutrient intake.

- Label and date all stored materials to monitor freshness.
- Combine multiple components for synergistic health effects, but adjust for individual tolerance.
- Maintain hygiene and safe handling to prevent contamination and preserve bioactive compounds.

Glossary

BIOACTIVE COMPOUNDS: Naturally occurring chemical constituents in plants, such as polyphenols, flavonoids, and medium-chain triglycerides, that exert biological effects on the body.

Cocos nucifera L.: The scientific name for the coconut plant, a tropical palm species valued for its nutritional, medicinal, and functional properties.

Decoction: A method of extraction in which plant materials (leaves, bark, roots) are boiled in water to release soluble bioactive compounds.

Functional Foods: Foods that provide additional health benefits beyond basic nutrition, often enriched with bioactive compounds to support specific physiological functions.

Herbal Extracts: Concentrated preparations derived from plant components, used for therapeutic or wellness purposes.

Holistic Wellness: An approach to health that integrates physical, mental, and social well-being, often incorporating nutrition, medicinal plants, lifestyle, and environmental considerations.

Medium-Chain Triglycerides (MCTs): A type of fat found in coconut oil and kernel that is rapidly metabolized for energy and may support metabolic health.

Nutraceuticals: Products derived from food sources that offer additional health benefits beyond basic nutrition, often in concentrated forms such as capsules, powders, or beverages.

Topical Application: The external use of plant-based preparations (oils, pastes, creams) on skin, hair, or nails for therapeutic or cosmetic purposes.

Decoction vs. Infusion: Decoction involves boiling plant materials for extraction, while infusion involves steeping in hot water for a shorter duration to preserve delicate bioactive compounds.

Phytonutrients: Naturally occurring plant chemicals, including antioxidants, flavonoids, and polyphenols, that support health and prevent disease.

Synergistic Combinations: The strategic integration of multiple plant components or nutrients to enhance overall health effects beyond individual contributions.

Sustainability: Practices that ensure the responsible utilization of natural resources, minimizing waste and environmental impact, often including full use of plant components.

Topical Paste: A semi-solid mixture of plant extracts and carrier substances (e.g., coconut oil) applied externally for therapeutic or protective effects.

Electrolyte Replenishment: Restoration of essential minerals such as potassium, sodium, and magnesium, often through consumption of coconut water or similar beverages.

Functional Preparations: Plant-based formulations, including teas, decoctions, smoothies, or topical applications, designed to deliver targeted health benefits.

Cultural and Traditional Knowledge: Information, practices, and beliefs about plant use passed through generations, often informing the selection and application of coconut components in nutrition and medicine.

Circular Economy: A sustainability model that emphasizes the full utilization of resources, minimizing waste, and creating value-added products from by-products.

Holistic Nutrition Plan: A structured approach to integrating diverse plant-based foods and preparations into daily routines to support systemic health and well-being.

Electrolytes: Minerals in bodily fluids that regulate physiological processes such as hydration, nerve function, and muscle contraction, commonly replenished by coconut water.

Topical Hydration: The application of oils or plant pastes on skin or hair to maintain moisture, protect tissue integrity, and support healing.

References

Abeywardena, M. Y., & Patten, G. S. (2011). Coconut oil and cardiovascular health: The potential role of medium-chain fatty acids. Nutrition Reviews, 69(6), 276–283. https://doi.org/10.1111/j.1753-4887.2011.00392.x

DebMandal, M., & Mandal, S. (2011). Coconut (Cocos nucifera L.): In health promotion and disease prevention. Asian Pacific Journal of Tropical Medicine, 4(3), 241–247. https://doi.org/10.1016/S1995-7645(11)60078-3

Henrietta, H. M., Kalaiyarasi, K., & Raj, A. S. (2022). Coconut tree (Cocos nucifera) products: A review of global cultivation and its benefits. Journal of Sustainability and Environmental Management, 1(2), 257–264. https://doi.org/10.3126/josem.v1i2.45377

Lima, E. B. C., Sousa, C. N. S., Meneses, L. N., Ximenes, N. C., Santos Júnior, M. A., Vasconcelos, G. S., Lima, N. B. C., Patrocínio, M. C. A., Macedo, D., & Vasconcelos, S. M. M. (2015). Cocos nucifera (Arecaceae): A phytochemical and pharmacological review. Brazilian Journal of Medical and Biological Research, 48(11), 953–964. https://doi.org/10.1590/1414-431X20154773

Marina, A. M., Che Man, Y. B., & Amin, I. (2009). Virgin coconut oil: Emerging functional food oil. Trends in Food Science & Technology, 20(10), 481–487. https://doi.org/10.1016/j.tifs.2009.06.003

Nadila, E., Azzahro, F., Yulisa Hasanah, F., & Proverawati, A. (2022). Composition and potency of young coconut water for health (Cocos nucifera L.): A systematic review. International Journal of Biomedical Nursing Review, 1(1), 10–18. https://doi.org/10.20884/1.ijbnr.2022.1.1.6528

Nevin, K. G., & Rajamohan, T. (2010). Effect of topical application of virgin coconut oil on skin components and antioxidant status during dermal wound healing in young rats. Skin Pharmacology and Physiology, 23(6), 290–297. https://doi.org/10.1159/000313516

Roshni, P., Bansod, S., Aswar, U., Akotkar, L., Kulkarni, V., & Shete, S. (2021). Pharmacological activities of coconut in metabolic diseases: A review. Journal of Phytopharmacology, 10(6), 478–483. https://phytopharmajournal.com/assets/pdf_files/Vol10_Issue6_08.pdf[1]

Shayanthavi, S., Kapilan, R., & Wickramasinghe, I. (2025). A comprehensive review of coconut liquid endosperm (Cocos nucifera L.): Composition, physicochemical characteristics, antimicrobial and antioxidant properties, and applications in microbial and tissue culture media. Journal of Science of the University of Kelaniya, 18(1), 1–18. https://doi.org/10.4038/josuk.v18i1.8119

Tuba, M., Olayinka, A., & Okonkwo, C. (2020). Nutritional and health benefits of coconut water and oil: A scientific review. African Journal of Food Science, 14(4), 91–99. https://doi.org/10.5897/AJFS2020.1912

Vijayakumar, S., Vasudevan, V., & Nair, R. (2019). Antioxidant and antimicrobial properties of Cocos nucifera oil and its fractions. Journal of Food Biochemistry, 43(3), e12779. https://doi.org/10.1111/jfbc.12779

1. https://phytopharmajournal.com/assets/pdf_files/Vol10_Issue6_08.pdf?utm_source=chatgpt.com

Don't miss out!

Visit the website below and you can sign up to receive emails whenever Mogana S. Flomo, Jr. publishes a new book. There's no charge and no obligation.

https://books2read.com/r/B-A-JCHY-OGMNH

Did you love *The Coconut Plant: Pathways to Health and Wellness*? Then you should read *Food and Drug Interactions: A Guide for the Health worker and Patient*[2] by Mogana S. Flomo, Jr.!

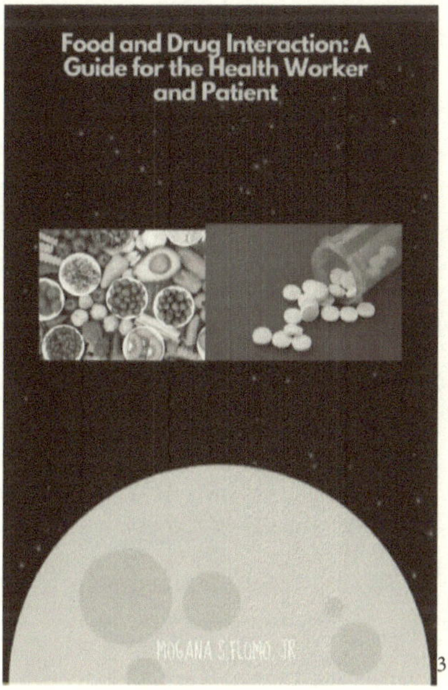

[3]

Food and drug interactions can occur when certain foods, drinks, or dietary supplements interfere with the way medications are absorbed, metabolized, or eliminated from the body. This can cause medications to be less effective, or it can increase the risk of side effects and adverse reactions. In this context, this book aims to provide readers with a comprehensive understanding of food and drug interactions and how to identify and avoid them. The book covers a range of topics, including common drug-nutrient interactions, how to read food and medication labels, the importance of talking to a healthcare provider, and sample meal plans for patients taking specific medications.

2. https://books2read.com/u/bOP6e0

3. https://books2read.com/u/bOP6e0

Additionally, the book offers practical tips and resources for patients and healthcare providers to help them navigate drug and food interactions effectively.

Also by Mogana S. Flomo, Jr.

First Edition

Introduction to University Studies

Rethinking PhD Training: A 21st Century Approach

HERBAL HEALTH

The Miracle of Bryophyllum pinnatum

The Coconut Plant: Pathways to Health and Wellness

Standalone

Food and Drug Interactions: A Guide for the Health worker and Patient

A Comprehensive Guide to Food Supplements

Collaboration and Knowledge Sharing in Armyworm Management

The Impact of Malaria on the Social-Economic Development of West Africa

Transforming Healthcare: Understanding Mobile Health Services in Underdeveloped Nations

Sustainable Approaches for Bird Conservation in Rice Farming: A Comprehensive Guide

Over-the-Counter (OTC) Medications: Your Comprehensive Guide to Safe and Effective Self-Care
Rejection: Embracing It and Using It
Understanding Environmental and Public Health Laws in Liberia
Understanding the National Commission on Higher Education in Liberia
School Human Resource Management
Gateways to Tomorrow: The Ultimate Admissions Guide
Integrated Disease Surveillance and Response (IDSR) in Africa
A Democratic Government: Understanding the System and Its Interconnected Parts
Short Notes On Water And Sanitation Management
Blacology

www.ingramcontent.com/pod-product-compliance
Lightning Source LLC
LaVergne TN
LVHW090422210926
848480LV00002B/649
* 9 7 9 8 2 3 2 5 5 8 8 0 2 *